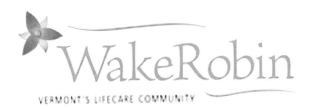

VERMONT'S LIFECARE COMMUNITY

This book is a gift
from the
Transitions Committee of the
Wake Robin Residents Association.

OUR LAST SIX MONTHS

AN ILLUSTRATED MEMOIR ABOUT DEATH,
CANCER, END-OF-LIFE CARE,
LOVE, FAMILY, AND
FORGIVENESS

by
Emily Bracale

ISBN: 978-1-947758-03-2

Produced by Maine Authors Publishing
12 High Street, Thomaston, ME 04861
www.maineauthorspublishing.com

Printed in the United States of America

To Aubrey,
with love always

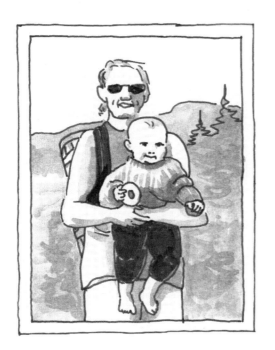
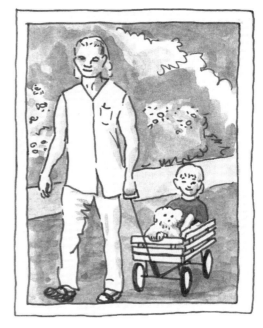
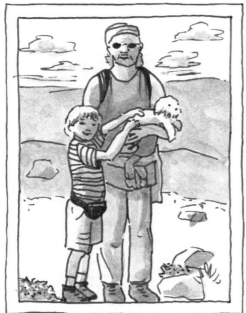
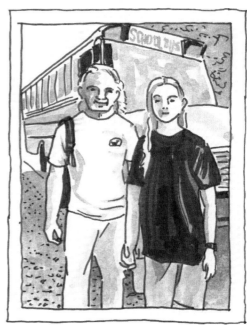

Preface and Thanks

For the past eight months, since my son's dad died of cancer, I've been working on this book. My utter delight and involvement in the process has made for some eyebrow-raising moments as people have offered their condolences. I have thanked them—and in the next breath informed them that I've been working on a sort of *comic* book about it! Let me explain where I'm coming from, and I think you'll see why this makes sense.

During the months before Aubrey's death, when I was helping him, my mind became too burdened and my attention span became too short to digest nonfiction books or lengthy novels, but when there was time to relax, then graphic novels and graphic memoirs kept my attention positively riveted. Some were about lovely things such as weddings and travel, but most were about serious things such as illness, cancer, death, and end-of-life care. Pictures made these subjects more approachable, and reading about other people's real-life challenges gave me more courage and perspective to deal with our situation. One day, I thought, I might create such a book about us: an ordinary family going through extraordinary circumstances. This idea didn't come out of the blue.

Since elementary school I've been journaling, painting, and making simple line drawings about daily life, so I was already taking notes and drawing a few cranky little comics in the midst of helping Aubrey—partly as a coping device. ("Gallows Humor" and "The Pants" are examples.) The inspiration and intention to actually get on with creating this book arrived during my drive to the crematorium. Suddenly I envisioned what it could be: a book I would have wanted to read even while down in the depths. I wanted so much to read it that I had to get on with making it! This project also assisted with the grieving process. It was both the method of digestion and the imperative to digest; I had to revisit what I'd been through and witnessed, then decide what to depict and describe. It turned out to have more text than a typical graphic memoir, several artistic styles instead of one, and lots of little themes within each chapter. While it is a real-life story, I did employ some poetic and artistic license to make the pieces hang together as a whole, and I altered some appearances, places, and names.

My hope is that this book will offer information, insights, comfort, and even laughter to other people, and help them become more prepared (or at least know they are not alone) should they ever have to face similar circumstances. I hope it sparks conversations about end-of-life choices, health care, and the medical insurance industry in this country. Beyond its focus on dying, this story is meant to be a celebration of Aubrey's life, and I hope that it offers some closure for his many loving fans who never had a chance to say good-bye.

Thanks to everyone who sent love and prayers and made donations to Aubrey's fundraiser; it would take a page of fine print to list everyone who helped us. Hospice's support was one of the brightest lights in the darkness, and I hope this story conveys my gratitude and encourages other families to seek what Hospice offers (that is, when the time comes). Thanks to my supreme editor Arthur Westing for such meticulous service. (Any remaining errors are my own.) Thanks to Steve Bohrer for all the loving encouragement through this difficult year, for always being supportive about this project, and for assisting in the polishing. Many thanks to all family members and friends who are represented as characters, especially my son, who showed interest in each new illustration, offered feedback on the writing, brought up more Dad stories, and was enthusiastic and willing to have me share them with the world. I offer these efforts with love and gratitude.

Emily Bracale
December 16, 2017

Main Characters

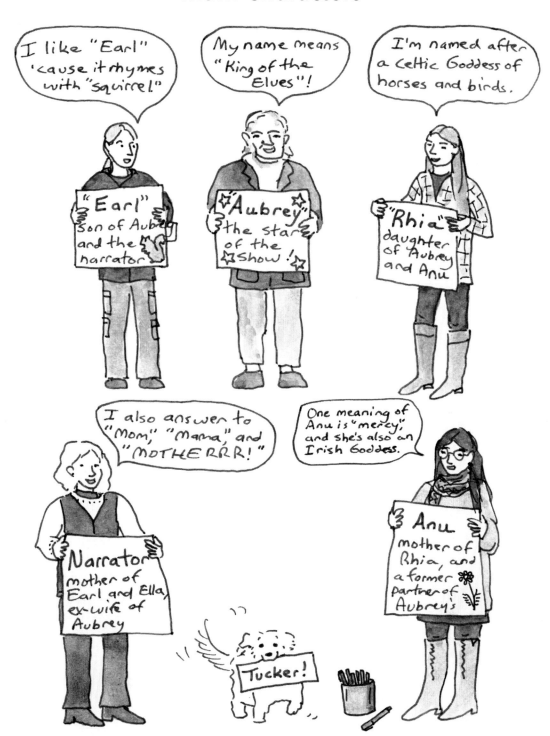

Complete List of Characters

FAMILY

The Narrator - mother of Earl and Ella, an ex-wife of Aubrey
Aubrey - father of Rhia and Earl
Earl - son of Aubrey and The Narrator
Ella - sister of Earl, daughter of The Narrator & The Gardener
Rhia - daughter of Aubrey and Anu
Anu - mother of Rhia, a former partner of Aubrey
Mark & Betty - Aubrey's brother and sister-in-law
Mumsie & Grand Pops - grandparents of Ella & Earl
The Gardener - Ella's dad, an ex-husband of The Narrator
Tucker - the little dog

FRIENDS

Steve - boyfriend of The Narrator
Landlord Lady (aka L.L.) - Aubrey's landlady
Nurse Bea - Aubrey's friend
The Turbanator - computer whiz, yoga teacher, Aubrey's friend
Moe - retired professor, founder of the Super Soup Kitchen
The Farmer - Aubrey's friend
Carpenter Man - Aubrey's friend

PROFESSIONALS

Aladdin - cancer survivor, food delivery volunteer
Angela - Hospital Clinical Social Worker
Helpful Hazel - Hospital Social Worker
Heliotrope - Hospital Case Manager
Mrs. Diplomacy - Hospital Patient Advocate
Dr. Kay - Aubrey's Primary Care Doctor
Dr. Spaceman - Aubrey's Oncologist
Nurse Spin - Oncology Nurse
Nurse Darlin' - Visiting Nurse
The Matron - Nursing Home Residential Care Director
The Cook - Nursing Home Dietitian

TABLE OF CONTENTS

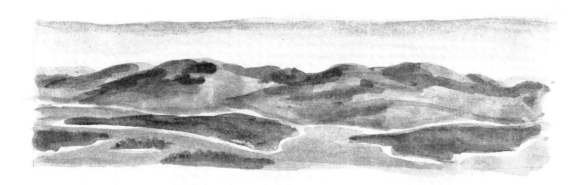

1.

As We Were

Dad Walks

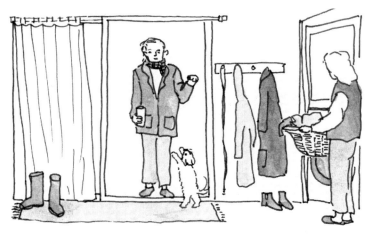
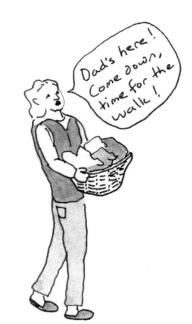

Every day, since Earl was born, his dad showed up for a walk.
Aubrey, my ex-husband, always knocked politely at my door.
Tucker, the little dog, was always happy to see him!

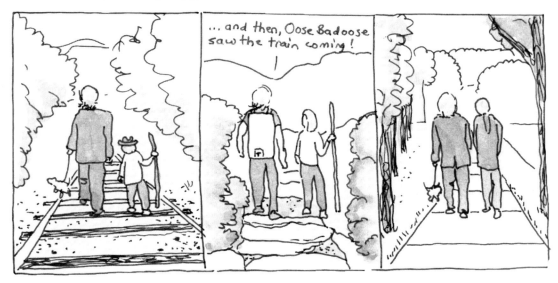

When Earl was quite young, his dad told him stories—incidents of mischief from his own childhood—playing with cousins in the country during summer vacations, sneaking over the fence into the baseball stadium near his house, and riding the rails by hopping freights.

Sometimes it was hard to tell what was for real and what was embellishment! His dad was a fine story teller.

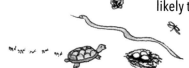

They were equally comfortable walking along in silence. Earl liked to daydream, and he knew if they were quiet they'd be more likely to encounter wild things.

12

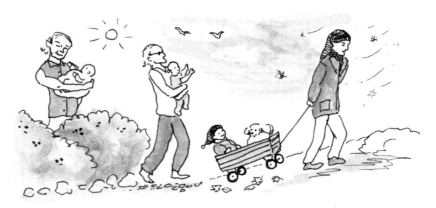

They went out walking in all kinds of weather. The only days that Aubrey missed were a blizzard, an ice storm, and whenever his car broke down.

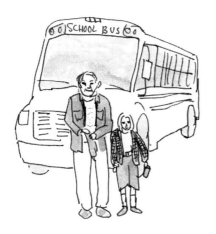

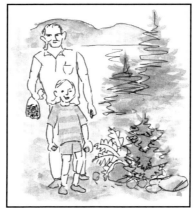

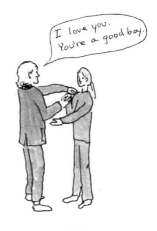

During the school year, Aubrey drove the morning bus route, went home to his apartment to write, then came to my house around lunch time. He worked at different schools, drove different routes in different years, but he always showed up for the Dad Walk.

Often he brought Earl a little treat: a freshly baked bagel with cream cheese from Agnes's bagel shop, or cookies, apples, and trail mix from the hiking camp he drove for every summer.

Every visit ended the same. Aubrey would say to his son, "I love you, you're a good boy." Then they would do their special handshake and one-armed casual guy hug.

After that, Aubrey went on to drive his afternoon bus route, then back to his apartment. I went back to solo parenting, being Head of Household, Self-employed, with one Dependent. It had been that way most of the time since Earl was born.

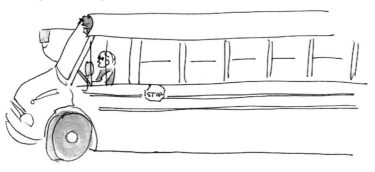

Home Economics

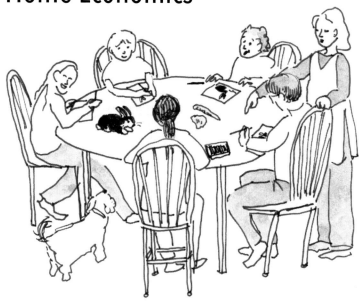

For earned income, May through October, I cleaned vacation rentals. The rest of the year I taught art classes around the dining room table, tutored students in reading, writing, and math, and occasionally met clients for Reiki and other healing support in my office upstairs. It wasn't a lot of income, but I got to claim Earl as a dependent on my taxes, so the refund helped us through the leaner months. Living under the poverty line, Earl and I both qualified for subsidized insurance, but Aubrey didn't until he turned sixty-five. Even then, Medicare didn't pay for all his medical bills or dental care—and his old car needed lots of maintenance. So, for the past couple of years, Child Support from him was low or nonexistent.

I didn't blame him. He lived as cheaply as a person could in this modern world. His wardrobe was built from clothing he found abandoned at the Lost & Found at the end of each school year, supplemented by pieces he bought at Goodwill. At least Earl got a little monthly payment of his own from the government when his dad became eligible for Social Security retirement benefits. By the time Earl was thirteen, his dad was sixty-seven.

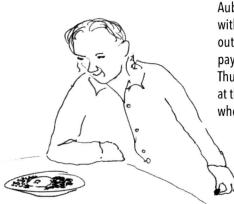

Sometimes he'd accept my invitation to stay for a meal with Earl and me after a walk.

(Tucker knew who to beg from at the table.)

Aubrey accepted his lot in life without complaining. If he ran out of money before his next pay check, he'd simply fast. On Thursdays he'd eat a big meal at the Super Soup Kitchen where he volunteered.

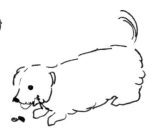

Occasionally he would ask me, with apologies, for a "cash transfusion" to put gas in his car.

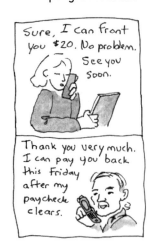

Sure, I can front you $20. No problem. See you soon.

Thank you very much. I can pay you back this Friday after my paycheck clears.

Earl lived with me full time, but once in a while Aubrey invited him out for burgers and fries, or to his apartment for dinner. They mostly ate the same four meals, adding broiled salmon as a special treat. Neither one minded this limited culinary pallet; in fact, both father and son thrived on predictability.

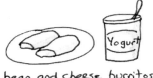

bean and cheese burritos with a dollop of yogurt

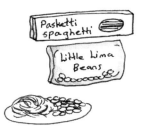

I wasn't much of a chef either, truth be known. Following detailed recipes wasn't my thing. Boxed macaroni and cheese, frozen peas, salad-in-a-bag, and canned soup were staples in my house. There were bulk bags of generic bean & cheese burritos in my freezer, too. Cooking fancy meals for one adult and one child was not my creative priority.

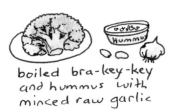

boiled bra-key-key and hummus with minced raw garlic

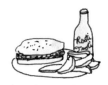

buffalo burger and home fries with root beer

Earl preferred to sleep at my house, in his own room, in his own bed, and his dad went along with that. So, after their dinners together, Aubrey always drove him back to my house for the night.

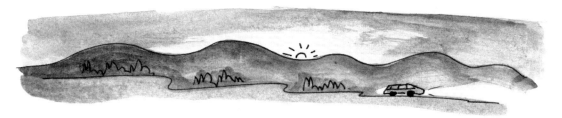

Occasionally, I wished for a night off, but I was happy to have Earl back in time for "cozy time." I loved to read aloud to him–picture books, fantasy fiction, Greek myths, Shakespeare's plays, political satire–and I could make sure his teeth were brushed, his hair was washed, his homework was finished, and so on.

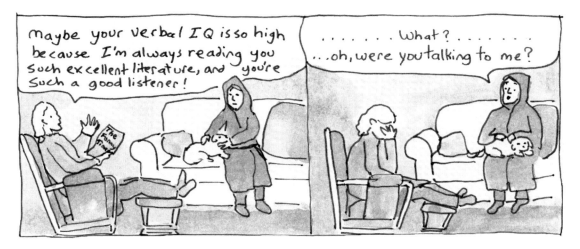

maybe your verbal IQ is so high because I'm always reading you such excellent literature, and you're such a good listener!

. . . . What? . . . .
...oh, were you talking to me?

Divorced Devotion

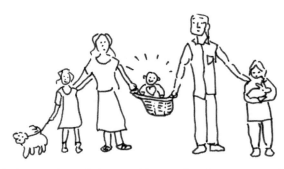

When Earl came along, Aubrey and I were already experienced parents. Earl had two half sisters: Aubrey's daughter Rhia, and my daughter Ella. Before he was born, the four of us lived under the same roof for several months. Aubrey and I were in amicable parenting partnerships with our daughters' other parents, or at least we all tried to be amicable, since we all lived in small communities close to one another.

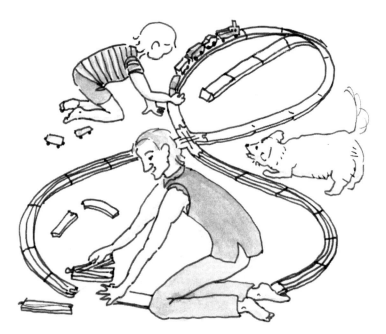

By the time Earl was born, Aubrey and I were separated, so Earl didn't ever spend much time with Rhia, and Ella was only there half the time. That, and the fact that his sisters were so much older than he was, meant Earl was virtually an only child in the way he was raised. He got a lot of one-on-one time with his dad and me. Having divorced older parents can have some advantages!

Besides coming over to take Earl on walks, Aubrey dedicated a lot of afternoons to watching over Earl and our neighbors' children as they played outside on our small town back street. He gave wagon rides, played catch, and helped them learn to ride bikes.

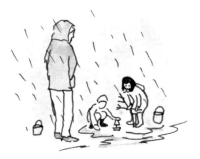

Whatever Earl found interesting, Aubrey patiently went along with. He never pressured Earl to play sports or perform or do whatever he himself had enjoyed as a child.

They shared a love of trains—the real, model, and toy kinds. Aubrey had fun getting down on the floor and constructing elaborate track layouts while Earl staged dramatic train crashes. Sometimes, to me, it looked like the "parallel play" of two children, each one independently focused on his own project, but content to be in the same room together.

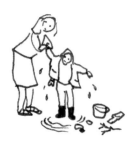

Although our relationship had been rocky at times, Aubrey and I kept renewing our vows to put our differences aside and put our son's needs first. We were devoted to being a functional parenting team.

If there were questions about Earl's health, we discussed them together. If he had interests he wanted to pursue, such as fencing and piano, we both supported him with our encouragement and cash as best we could. I paid for music lessons, and Aubrey paid for fencing lessons. When there were conferences and concerts at school, we attended them together, even if we arrived and left in separate cars.

After Earl did some testing at the end of third grade, home-schooling was highly recommended to meet his needs. By seventh grade he was also going up to the school for a few subjects. Sometimes Aubrey picked him up from a class before their walk, or dropped him off for an afternoon class on his way to his afternoon bus run. All I had to do was ask; Aubrey was always glad to help.

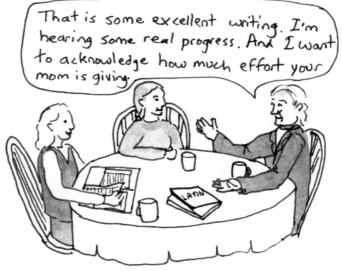

Each month we would meet as a family to praise Earl's accomplishments, encourage him with his challenges, and help him set new goals for the next month. Aubrey gave good pep talks, to Earl and also to me.

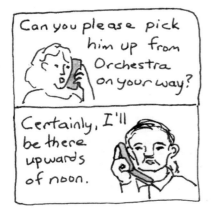

It had not always been so respectful between us. But for several years we had been "flying at cruising altitude," having transcended the turbulence. We had a basic functional routine, with enough peace and harmony—and so little drama—that had someone set out to write a book about us, it would have been fairly boring.

Our Supporting Cast

A few family members lived nearby. My daughter Ella, Earl's half sister, was attending college just up the road. She often popped over to join us for a meal. Sometimes she swooped up Earl for an overnight, during which they would discuss global issues and binge-watch sit-coms. Though they were eight years apart, they got along swimmingly. She was old enough to function as another adult in his life, treating him to Thai takeout and pizza deliveries, but she was also young enough to relish being silly.

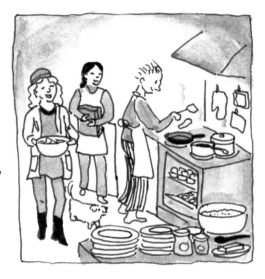

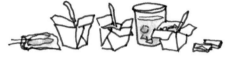

Her dad, The Gardener, also lived nearby. We got along well enough that I still did drawings for his business. He was very busy, and traveled a lot, but when he had time he invited Earl and me to join him and Ella for a meal. He had come to accept Aubrey, on account of caring for Earl, and often told Earl how lucky he was to have Aubrey for a dad.

Now and then Ella's college friends initiated a Sunday brunch. I was happy to provide the full kitchen for them to play in, the cozy living room with a fireplace, and to be served, for a change!

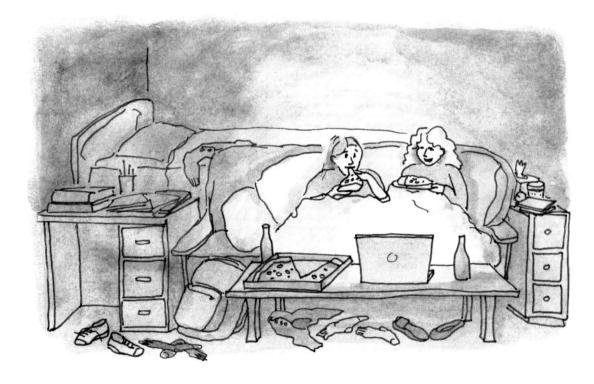

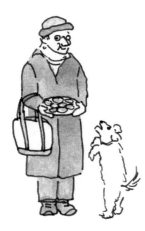

My parents, known to my children as "Mumsie and Grand Pops," lived close by in the countryside. They came to our house every Friday afternoon, often bearing gluten-free cookies. They kindly took our garbage to the dump along with theirs, then came back to read aloud in the living room. It was a sweet way to end the school week. I would make them weak decaf coffee, affectionately known as "Mumsie water," and join in the listening.

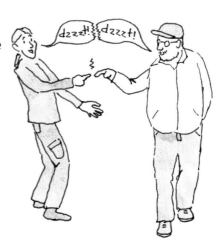

Back in the early days of Earl's life they lived in another state, so we only saw them twice a year. Their opinion of Earl's dad was not very high at times, but since the winter they had moved close by they'd gotten to know him better and now regarded him with affection. Sometimes they invited him over for coffee, and they were another source of short-term loans when they could not help noticing the balding tires on his old car or his need for winter boots.

They recognized in him a fellow animal lover who would go out of his way to lift a turtle off the road or carry a spider outdoors. So, lucky for me, when they went on overnight trips to see my sister and her family far away, he would house-sit their cats. These cats were very old, and the cat box needed frequent cleaning. One of them took a liking to the blanket Aubrey used during his morning meditation and yoga, so he left the blanket at their house for the cat.

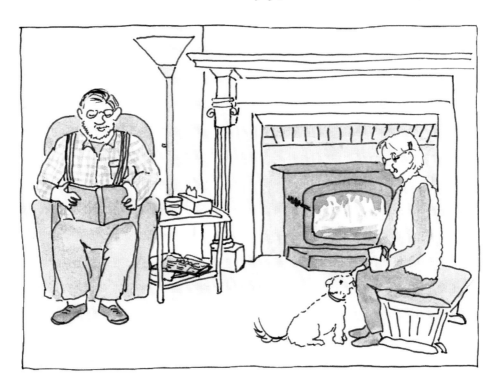

My boyfriend, Steve, had a good job at a good college in The Big City. He drove up two or three weekends a month and stayed longer for some vacations.

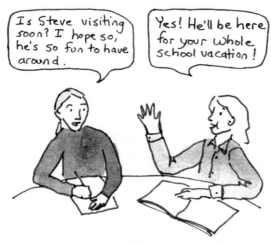

He and Earl had been buddies ever since their first sword fight. Steve was just a friend of the family then, staying at our house as a guest while he was in town to see his own daughter over the holidays.

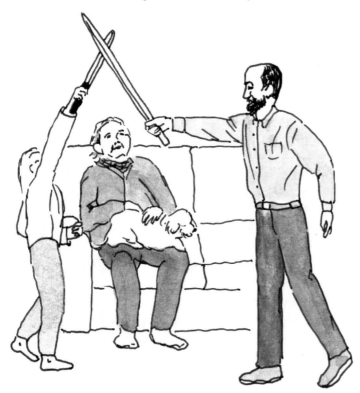

Steve got along with everyone, including both of my ex-husbands. He was easy-going, clever with words, and very tall and handsome. When Steve and I started dating, Aubrey said, "Steve is a good man. You couldn't ask for a better man than Steve." (I was, naturally, grateful for his endorsement.)

Steve respected Aubrey as Earl's dad, and never attempted to act parental with Earl himself–aside from a few tips on table manners, bike riding, and how to use hand tools and swear effectively. To Earl he became a "favorite uncle" sort of figure.

Although ours was a long-distance relationship, we felt so at home with one another that it was always a pleasure, like dancing.

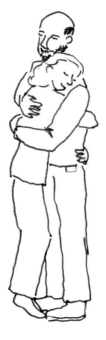

To our advantage, starting out, we had almost two decades of friendship, and mutual admiration for one another as professionals and former colleagues.

Occasionally I asked Ella or my mother to stay at my house with Earl, and I would make the five hour trip out of state to visit Steve at his apartment in The Big City.

Earl and I also had friends, neighbors, and a few other family members who visited once in a while. But our daily life revolved around home-schooling, working from home, Ella dropping by alone or with her friends, the Grand Parental Units making their weekly rounds, Steve providing a happy break two or three weekends a month, and daily visits with Aubrey. Life went on like this for long enough that we were all used to it.

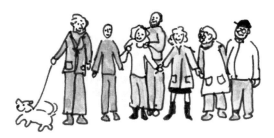

My health was not spectacular, but living a simple life suited me fine. Aspirations for career ladder climbing or further degree earning or adventurous world traveling were over. I aspired to live within my means and take responsibility for what was mine to care for: son, dog, house, work, myself. Beyond part-time jobs, I considered it a good day if I managed to feed Earl and myself three meals, drive him to lessons on time, teach him some new spelling words and Algebra, feed the dog, take a hot bath, and still have energy to read a book or watch a movie in bed.

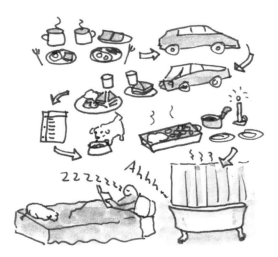

If I wanted to kick things up a notch, I might open a bottle of Merlot and pour half a glass to sip along with the movie, or watch sci-fi instead of a rom-com.

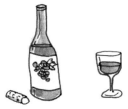

Earl seemed content, for the most part, to have evenings to himself: reading a fantasy fiction novel, playing computer games, and maybe doing a bit of sketching, wood carving, or metalwork in the base-ment. Sometimes we watched a or history documen-tary together and shared a bowl of popcorn.

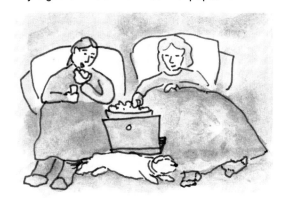

We had no idea what lay ahead of us in the New Year. If some psychic had predicted our future, we would have run screaming in the opposite direction...

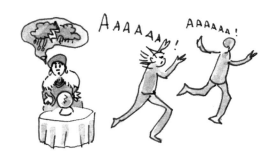

...or, simply rolled our eyes in disbelief.

2.

The Beginning of the End

Study Hall

Late in the year in which Earl turned thirteen, the Dad Walks got shorter and shorter, often just a stroll around the block. In December, the two of them switched to reading and writing, side by side, in the living room. Aubrey brought his computer. Earl read a novel or did workbooks. As with their walks, they didn't talk much. They called this hour "Study Hall."

Earl sat on the blue couch with the dog, and Aubrey sat in the Dad Chair, which looked a bit throne-like with its rich red upholstery marbled with gold.

While they had Study Hall, I would go out and do chores, making the rounds in our small town which had a bakery, grocery store, bank, library, post office, YMCA, and hospital, all within three blocks of my house. In good weather I'd walk or ride my bike, but in December I drove because it was always cold and wet outside.

The dog didn't like getting wet, and only wanted short walks anyway, so rainy weather partially masked the fact that walks stopped because of Aubrey's declining health. But Earl and I had noticed some subtle changes in him, such as the way he was becoming stiff in the knees. I thought that was arthritis, old age setting in. He was sixty-seven, after all. Then, uncharacteristically, he stopped drinking coffee, and when I offered him Mumsie's gluten-free cookies he declined. He explained that he had a gum infection and was trying to avoid sugar. He said he was on a liquid diet of high-protein smoothies and special vitamins and herbal supplements.

Earl and his dad discussed the problem of the stiff knees: if the rain and sleet ever turned to snow, might they go cross-country skiing instead of walking? Would that be gentler on Aubrey's knees? He declared he would indeed like to try that, and maybe buy himself cross-country skis, some day. (Later, Earl and I discussed this, and made a secret plan to pool our resources and buy his dad skis for Christmas.)

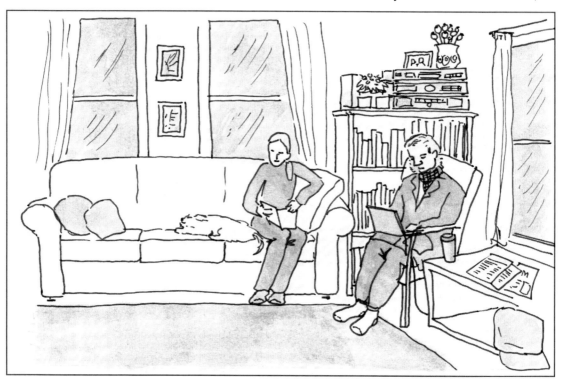

Becoming Prepared

I don't know if I would go so far as to call it a "Divine Plan" or a "Compassionate Universe," but looking back, I can see how several events (and non-events) helped me to be at least somewhat prepared for what happened in the New Year.

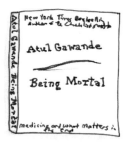

Clue #1: Reading the book *Being Mortal*, by Atul Gawande. My mother discovered it through a book group at the library. As a former nurse, she appreciated Dr. Gawande's perspective on end-of-life care, and his critique of our country's provisions for its elderly. She hoped my father would read it too, so they could consider some of the choices and issues it raised, but he stopped at page 65. So I started reading it, just to be nice to her, but then I was glad; we had some honest talks about our own preferences regarding end-of-life care and other issues the book described.

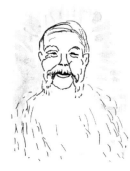

Clue #2: Dreaming of a grateful dead man. The last time this client came for Reiki, I knew he was very ill, and I didn't know if I would ever see him again. He went for some tests, his cancer had come back, and soon he was in the hospital. A few weeks later, he appeared to me in a dream, with a big smile on his face, telling me he was glad to feel all better! I could hardly believe it! But he smiled again, reassuringly. A couple of days later I found out that he had died that night. When I shared the dream and his message with his wife, she was also grateful. We both believed in some kind of life after death—a spiritual reality, at least—beyond the mortal body. We both found the dream reassuring.

Clue #3: Taking a two-hour Ayervedic health workshop, focused on self-care in the wintertime. I wanted to be more prepared to thrive (instead of merely survive) five months of cold soggy harsh gloomy weather.

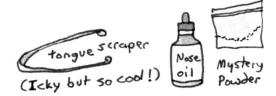

tongue scraper (Icky but so cool!) Nose oil Mystery Powder

Clue #4: No work lined up for the winter! In spite of advertising, even with happy former clients spreading word through the grapevine, I had no new art or tutoring gigs lined up for the New Year. After the holidays, other than Earl's class and lesson schedule, my calendar was blank.

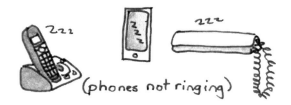

(phones not ringing)

Clue #5: Deciding to rent out a room. During the past year I had earned so little money from Reiki that I concluded my home office would be more lucrative as a student rental. I planned to put up an ad at the college when the new term started in January.

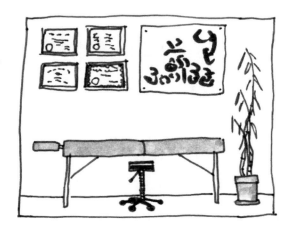

Movies and Cocoa

Aubrey told Earl and me that he would be away at Christmas, for the first time ever. He would be driving out of state to see his daughter, Rhia. It would be her first Christmas away from home because of her new job. She had recently graduated from college. Earl and I had not seen her in years. Aubrey would be driving down with Rhia's mom, Anu, who lived about a forty minutes away.

We decided we could celebrate Christmas with him when he got back. Before he went away, however, he brought up the special ritual he and Earl partook of annually.

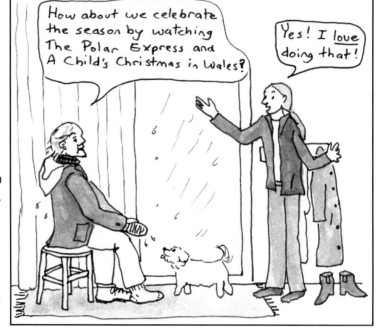

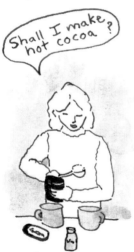

I knew my part in the ritual. Few things are as cozy as hot cocoa on a cold rainy day in December. I was surprised, but pleased, when Aubrey said yes. It made everything feel normal again.

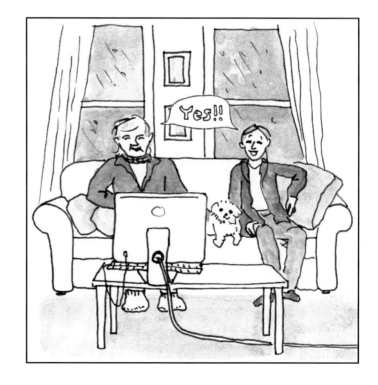

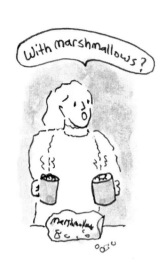

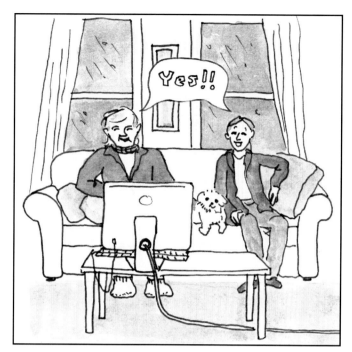

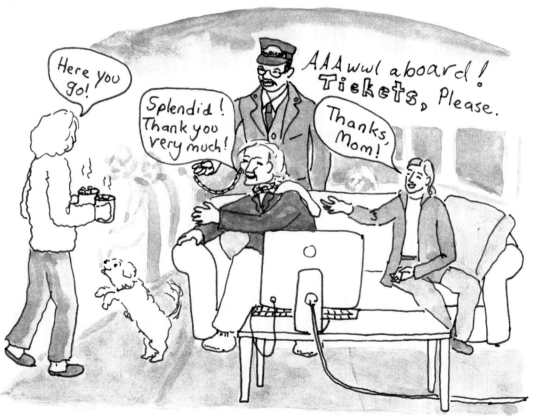

The Lump

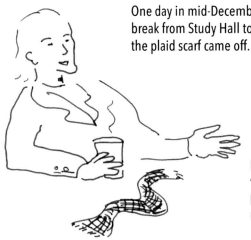

One day in mid-December, when Aubrey took a break from Study Hall to have a hot cup of tea, the plaid scarf came off.

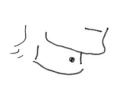

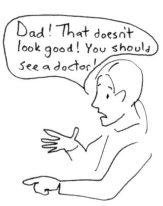

Dad! That doesn't look good! You should see a doctor!

Earl and I saw the lump.
"What is that, Dad?"
It looked like a growth of some kind...
I think we all knew what it was, but we didn't name it.

Aubrey explained that he was taking homeopathic, herbal, and Ayervedic medicines, and that these natural treatments worked slowly–one needed to be patient–but he felt confident they would help.
Perhaps they would, but were they enough, soon enough?
When does do-it-yourself treatment become less useful?
Had he been making an effort to hide it all along?
He was being brave to endure hard times,
and had a strong will, for better or for worse.
As his ex-wife, it wasn't my role to question his self-care plan.
But I did strongly suggest that he get the lump biopsied right away.
In my mind I saw images of taking care of him when he would need help.

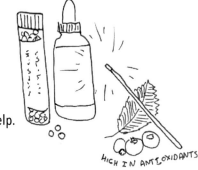

HIGH IN ANTIOXIDANTS

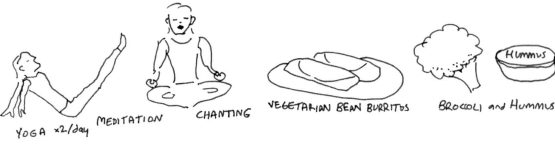

YOGA x2/day   MEDITATION   CHANTING   VEGETARIAN BEAN BURRITOS   BROCCOLI and HUMMUS

It was hard to conceive of Aubrey being ill. He had been one of the most healthy people I knew. No smoking or drinking, few desserts, a vegetarian diet (for the most part, camp picnics and Thanksgiving dinners aside). He ate lots of kale. He even saved and drank the water from the broccoli he boiled. Broccoli juice, yuck!

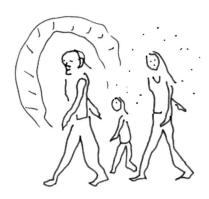
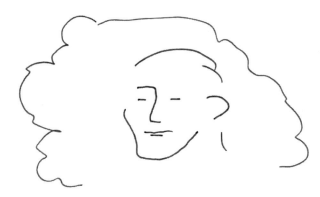

He hiked every day in summer.
He ate raw garlic almost every day.
Bugs never bit him.
He did not get colds or flu.

He did yoga daily at sunrise, and late in the afternoon. I'll never forget the first time I saw him doing a hand stand. We had just moved in together. I stood in the bedroom doorway, looking into the livingroom, in awe. His back was to me. I could see his arm muscles bulging. I could barely do a push-up. Would he think I was weak and flabby? Should I try to learn yoga to be better paired? Should I drink broccoli juice, too? I went back to correcting my students' papers and planning lessons. I heard his feet come back to the ground, then there was silence, for a long time. I thought he was meditating. It was almost dinnertime. I peeked my head back into the living room and found him sitting at the low coffee table, with the care package my mother had sent, eating the chocolate frosted chocolate date cookies.

"These are amazing!" he said, "You better take them away from me before I eat them all!"

Phew! We weren't so different, after all!

In terms of New Age spiritual beliefs about how to manifest good health, he was doing everything he could be doing. He meditated on peace and light and kept up a positive attitude. Every time anyone asked him how he was feeling, he'd say,

"Splendid!"

In terms of diet and exercise, he was a model to be admired. His friend Carpenter Man said Aubrey taught him so much about improving his own health through yoga, and that Aubrey was the real deal: a real yogi, dedicated to the practice, not just doing it because it was hip.

But in December, day by day, Aubrey's voice became more hoarse and gravelly. A new lump emerged by his upper lip. Earl and I noticed he was having a hard time putting his shoes back on after visits. The question that plagued us was: If such a person could become so sick, what chance did the rest of us have?

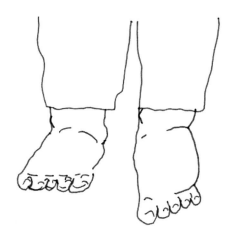

Diabetic Dog

The same week the lump was revealed, I took Tucker to the vet. He had been acting weirdly. The vet diagnosed that he had diabetes, and needed to be given insulin shots twice a day, twelve hours apart, for the rest of his life, starting immediately! I asked what would happen if we didn't treat him, if I could not manage all that. She was a bit taken aback! I quickly surrendered resistance and the mothering instinct kicked in: to do whatever it took. I learned how to monitor his blood glucose level and give him insulin shots.

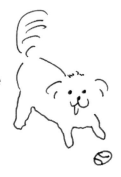

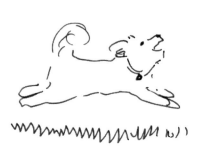

The dog was 12, going on 13, but still acted like a puppy when feeling well.

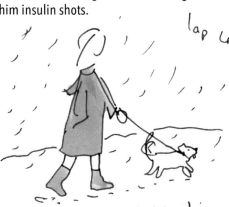

I started taking him out for walks, which did get me to go out more, as winter weather set in, so even though this was a new chore, it was beneficial as well.

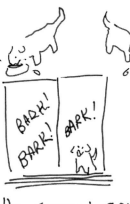

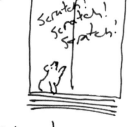

He seemed anxious to go outside all the time though.

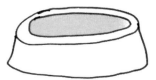

And went through big bowls of water very quickly. And peed all the time. And panted non stop, unless asleep.

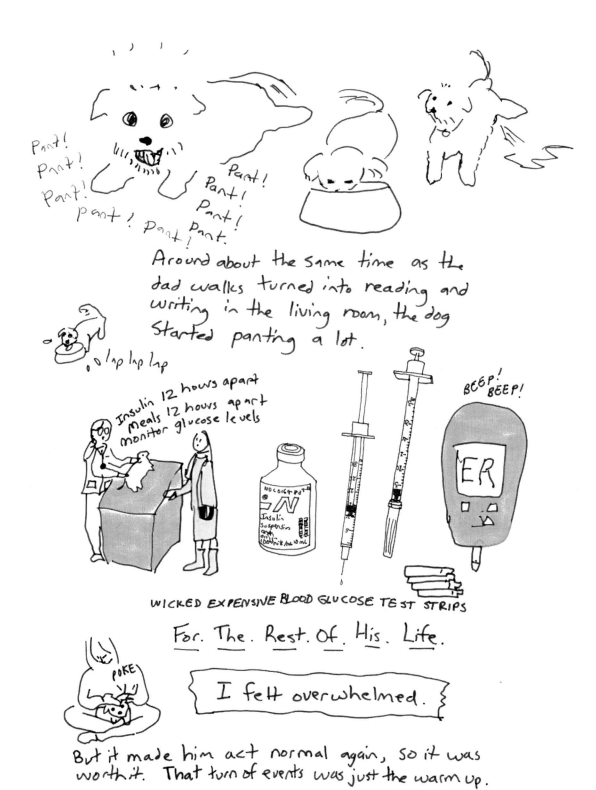

Pant! Pant! Pant! Pant! Pant! Pant! Pant! Pant!

Around about the same time as the dad walks turned into reading and writing in the living room, the dog started panting a lot.

lap lap lap

Insulin 12 hours apart
meals 12 hours apart
monitor glucose levels

NDC 0164-20

N

Insulin suspension

100 units/mL 10 mL

BEEP! BEEP!

ER

WICKED EXPENSIVE BLOOD GLUCOSE TEST STRIPS

For. The. Rest. Of. His. Life.

POKE

I felt overwhelmed.

But it made him act normal again, so it was worth it. That turn of events was just the warm up.

Festive Times

Earl and Ella decorated the Christmas tree. I used to do it, but was glad they took over. It looked so magical with the lights on and all the old special ornaments!

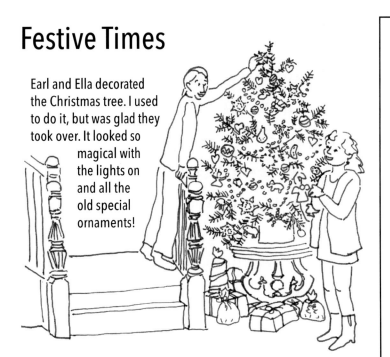

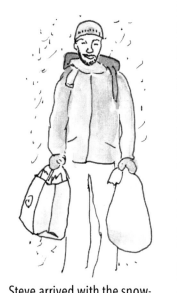

Steve arrived with the snow-storm. He was staying for two weeks! Vacation had begun!

Ella and I baked her dad's favorite holiday bread, potica ("po-ti-tza"), with walnut, raisin, and poppyseed filling.

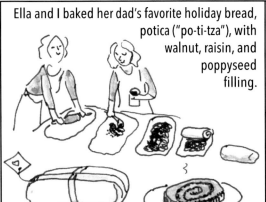

Everyone wrapped presents secretly.

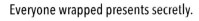
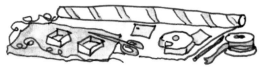

Steve and Earl shoveled snow.

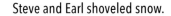

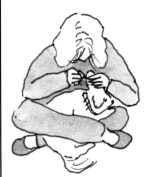

I poked Tucker's ears a lot in order to measure his blood glucose level. He finally resigned himself to the fact and stopped violently shaking his head.

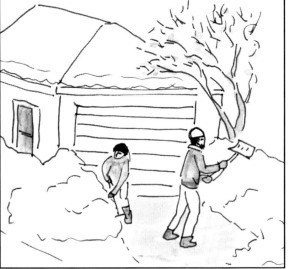

My sister and her family drove up from out of state. They stayed at Mumsie and Grand Pop's house and everyone came to my house to open presents on Boxing Day, the day after Christmas.

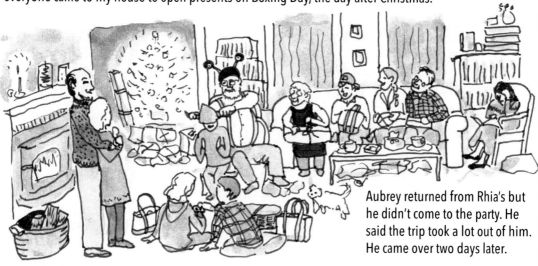

Aubrey returned from Rhia's but he didn't come to the party. He said the trip took a lot out of him. He came over two days later.

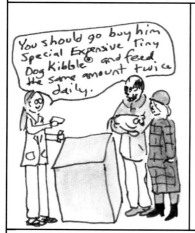

You should go buy him Special Expensive Tiny Dog Kibble® and feed the same amount twice daily.

Steve came with me to the vet. Having Type 1 Diabetes himself, he asked the vet good questions and he helped me understand about carbohydrates and blood glucose levels and insulin.

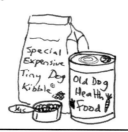

Earl gave his dad the skis.

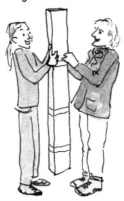

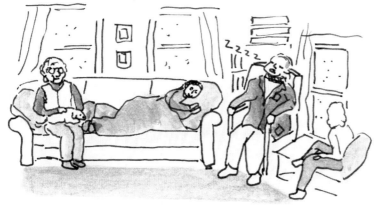

Grand Pops read aloud, Earl lounged on the blue couch, Aubrey stayed and enjoyed the family time, then nodded off and snored in his red and gold Dad Chair.

Mumsie and I exchanged glances.

The New Year Begins

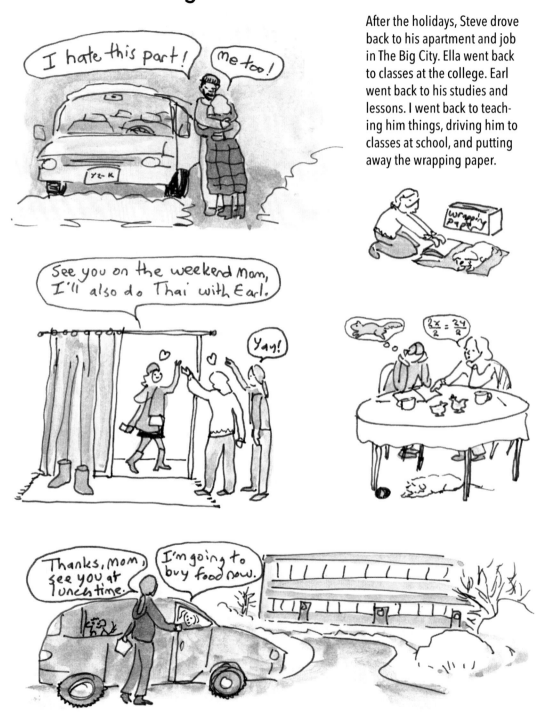

After the holidays, Steve drove back to his apartment and job in The Big City. Ella went back to classes at the college. Earl went back to his studies and lessons. I went back to teaching him things, driving him to classes at school, and putting away the wrapping paper.

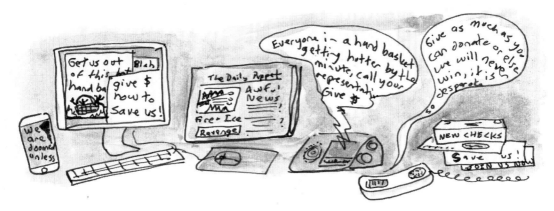

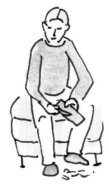

Outside the little bubble of our household, the national news was filled with dreadful stories and pictures, so much so that it was nerveracking to listen to the radio or read a newspaper. A sense of foreboding filled the air. I donated token amounts of money, made phone calls to my representatives, and prayed a lot. Handwork also helped: Earl carved wood, and I crocheted lots of hats.

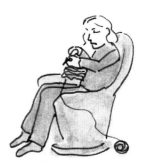

Aubrey went back to driving the school bus. But he complained about it more than ever: having to wake up and put gas in the bus before dawn, driving through freezing rain, backing into a ditch, and having to get the bus towed.

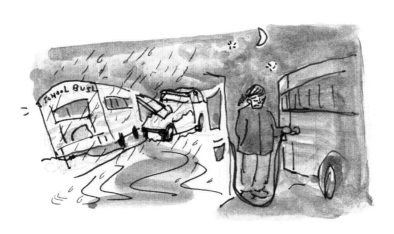

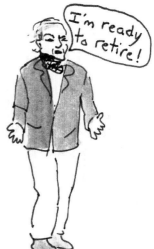

Finding Out

Monday, January 9th, Aubrey announced:

We sympathized. The job was too rough on him. His health came first. Money would work out somehow. Earl asked if he'd been to a doctor yet. Aubrey worked at his tight boots, then responded, calmly.

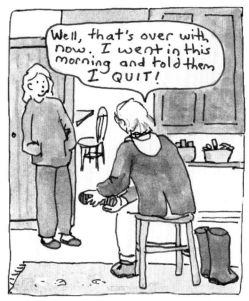

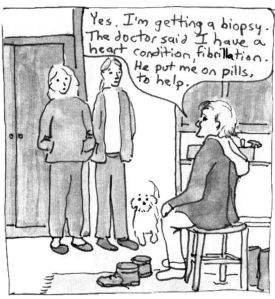

Well, a heart condition! That was news! And a decent excuse to retire. I remembered another time he had quit his bus job. We'd been married at the time. I'd supported him financially for a while, until it became untenable. At least this time he was old enough to be receiving Social Security retirement benefits.

I asked if he'd told anyone at work about his health, and he said no. I knew his aversion to official business, including filling out forms, so I offered to pick up a housing application and help him fill it out. There was a subsidized housing facility just up the street. He could walk here and Earl could walk there.

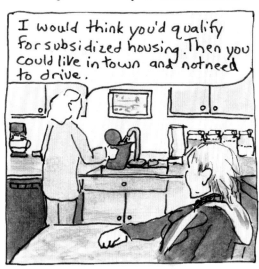

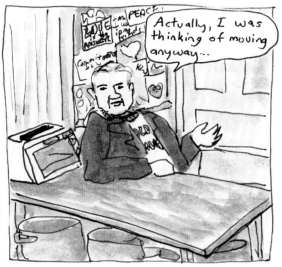

He explained that he wanted to change his diet, but his landlord was strictly vegan, because of her spiritual beliefs, and she didn't want any animal products to be served or consumed under her roof.

Tuesday, January 10th, we didn't see Aubrey because he had another appointment, and he didn't call after it to give us a report. We tried to be patient, but it was the only thing we could think about.

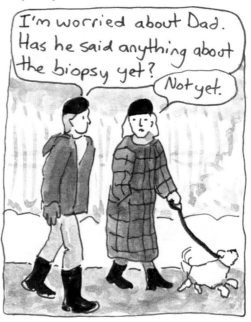

My doctor says I'm protien deficient. I want to start eating eggs and buffalo burgers, but she said I'll have to eat them elsewhere!

I'll pick up a housing application for you today!

I'm worried about Dad. Has he said anything about the biopsy yet?

Not yet.

Wednesday, January 11th, Aubrey picked Earl up from Social Studies, we all ate lunch (toast and eggs), then they had Study Hall. Aubrey filled out the housing application himself. Then he prepared to leave. I confronted him when Earl was out of hearing range.

I was confused. I thought the jaw was "just" a gum infection, and the biopsy was of the lump on the neck. But the mass in the jaw was a cancerous tumor. Melanoma. The lump on the neck must be also. I asked Aubrey if he wanted me to help him tell Earl.

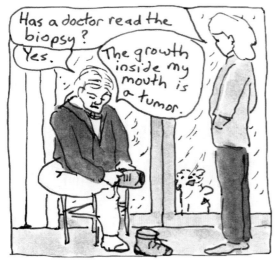

Has a doctor read the biopsy?

Yes.

The growth inside my mouth is a tumor.

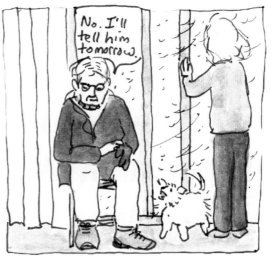

No. I'll tell him tomorrow.

I could have broken the news to Earl, myself, but I respected that it wasn't my news to tell. I told my parents, though, and they were not surprised. My mother said she had known people with cancer, and from what she observed, including his swollen feet and rapid decline, she didn't think he would live much longer, maybe a few months, or just weeks.

I stayed up all night writing and praying. I got some clear guidance of what to do and for about how long.

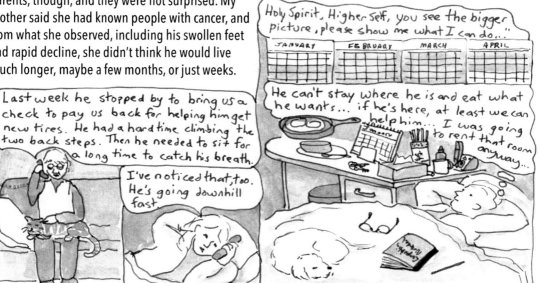

Thursday, January 12th, when Aubrey came over, I told him what I felt moved to offer, but I tried to put it to him carefully. He talked as if he were expecting to fully recover and be able to keep driving and living independently into the far future. If making my offer sound temporary helped him to accept help, so be it.

When Earl came home from French, Aubrey told him about the cancer. I was not in the living room at the time, so I don't know how it went. Later, I talked with Earl a bit. He was very sad, but realistic. He agreed that his dad should move in with us, at least temporarily. He understood that it was up to us to help.

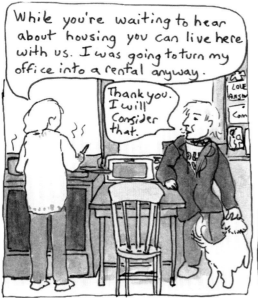

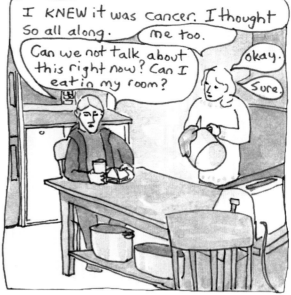

That evening I talked to Aubrey again, on the phone. He confided that he had known about the cancer for two years, and that it was melanoma. The question, "Why didn't you tell us?!" came to my mind.

When he explained the option his doctor had given him at the time, I realized his choice to keep the cancer a secret was his honorable effort to protect us from worrying about something we couldn't fix.

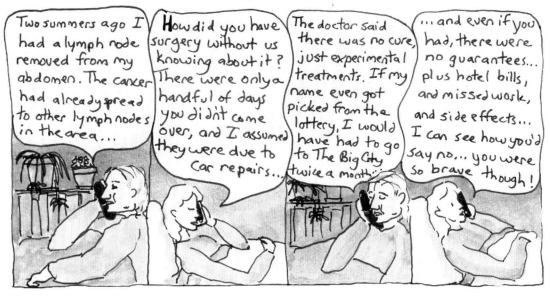

Knowing his reticence to upset anyone with bad news, I urged him to reach out and call Rhia and her mom right away. Now that Earl and I knew, it was only fair to let others in the family know so they didn't feel left out. He acknowledged the point.

Friday, January 13th, Aubrey said yes to moving in! I was so relieved! He assured me this would only be temporary, and he was most grateful. As I moved my belongings out of my office and made it into a bedroom, I felt it was absolutely the right thing to do.

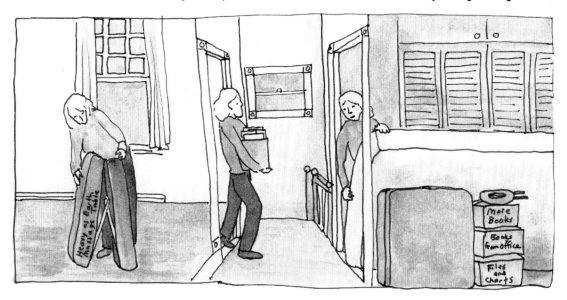

Going Out, Moving In

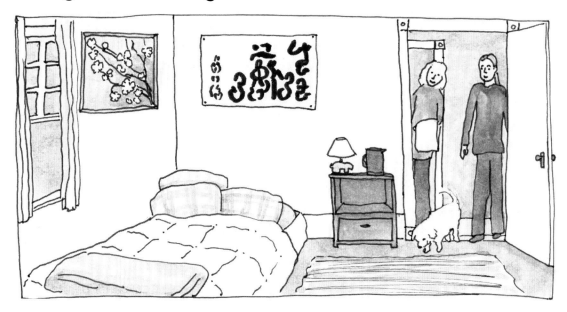

The finished guest room looked simple, cozy, and clean. If I thought of us as a divorced couple moving back in together, but in separate bedrooms, it felt strange. If I thought of us in a dormitory, where we each had our own sovereign quarters, our own privacy bubbles, it made sense. How would it feel? How long would it last?

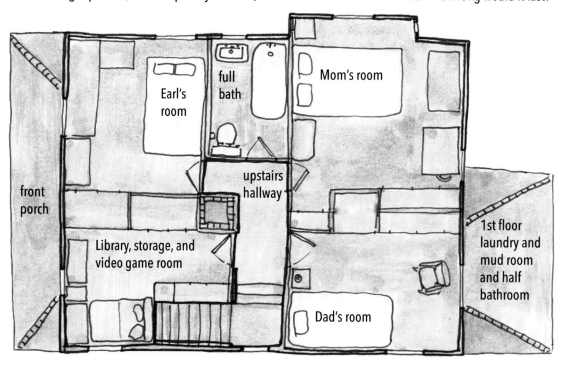

Saturday, January 14th, began happily. Steve had arrived late the night before. Earl and I were so glad to see him! He always brought levity. After we all slept in, we all went out to brunch. Our daughters met us at the restaurant. (This was a rare assemblage of characters, given their busy college schedules.) They had been friends since childhood, long before we'd started dating. We were "going steady" but had no plans to blend our families under one roof and no expectations for one another to act as a parent to our children. Our daughters had fledged already, anyhow. It was simply nice to all connect, once in a while, around a table, for a meal.

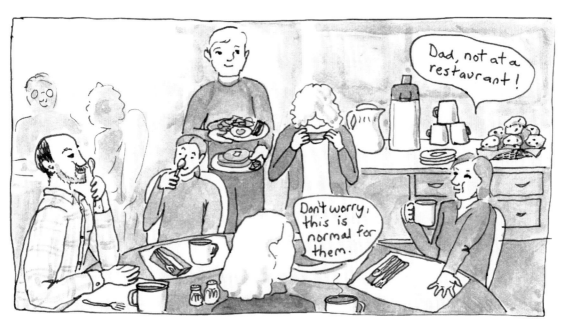

When we came home I called Aubrey to see if he needed help packing his belongings into his car. He said Landlord Lady and their mutual friend, Nurse Bea, were there helping him, and they had already done the lion's share. He was about ready to make the drive over! When he arrived, a half hour later, Steve and Earl and I helped carry his things into the house and up the stairs.

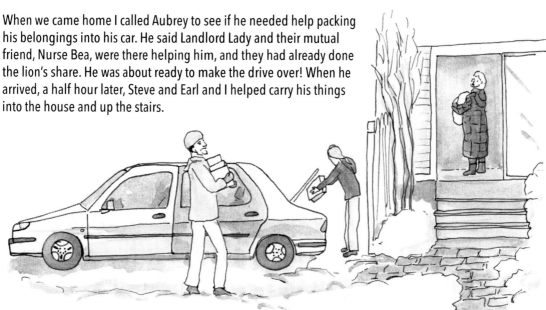

I held back most of the clothing in the laundry room as it smelled musty and I was very particular about such things. Other than that there were only some plants, his computer, two heavy dictionaries, some photo albums, food, papers, books, and countless bottles of supplements. Everything he owned fit into one carload.

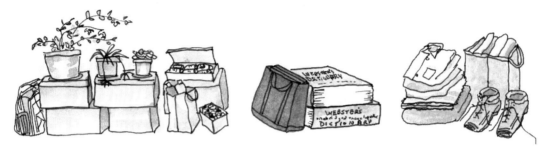

The man himself sat down in his chair in the living room, and caught his breath. When he was ready to tackle the stairs, he took them slowly. As I watched, from the living room, I wished I had a ground floor room to offer, but once he made it up to his room he could rest, and we could bring him meals on a tray, and the full bath was upstairs anyway. "Ah, the claw-footed tub! I will enjoy that!" he said.

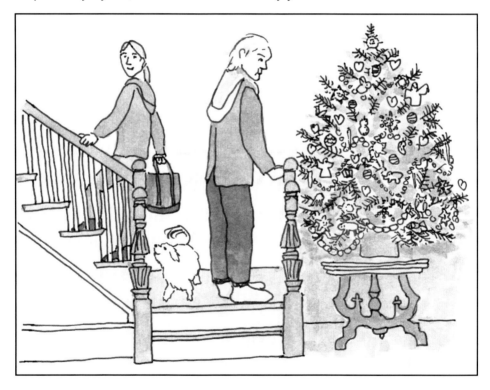

Earl brought Aubrey's black canvas bag with his laptop computer up to his room, that being the only material object to which Aubrey seemed attached. It held his work-in-progress, a novel of great mystery, which he had been working on daily for over a year. When he saw his room he was very grateful and pleased. He declared that the first order of business was a nap. Tucker curled up with him on the end of the futon. Aubrey wanted the door to be left open so he didn't feel claustrophobic, so the dog came and went as he pleased.

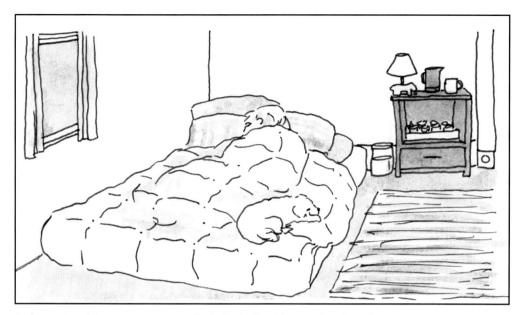

Earl went into his own room across the hall, closing his own door for privacy.
I went back downstairs to start the laundry.
Steve helped me find places for all the new food in the kitchen, and we made dinner together.
We could hear Aubrey snoring in the distance.
Earl brought him a dinner tray, for which he was most grateful.
After he ate, he slept some more.

As I cuddled in with Steve for the night, we discussed the situation. It was a lot to take in.
Everything felt new and different, yet also complete; as if everyone were in their right place in the world. Saturday, January 14th, ended cozily.

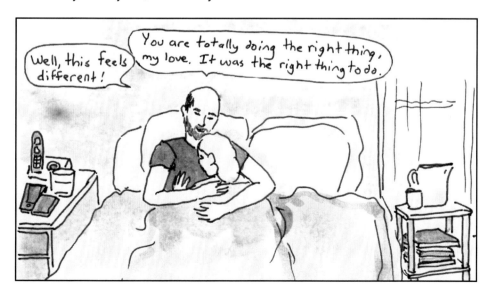

Healing Support

The next day Landlord Lady and Nurse Bea came by with a few more books and more jars and baggies of Aubrey's food from L.L.'s refrigerator. I felt a tiny bit annoyed about having to sort through, throw away, and make room for more of his old food.

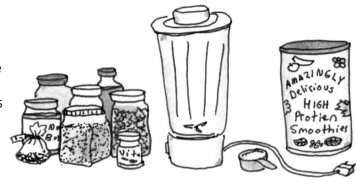

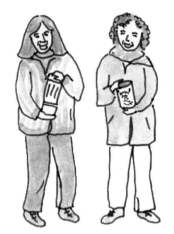

But they also came bearing two very useful gifts: a mini blender, and a canister of very expensive vegetarian smoothie powder, a kind that Aubrey especially liked.

Both of these women were among the interesting people I had gotten to meet through Aubrey, and they had known him for years before I met him. We all shared interests in spirituality and alternative and holistic healing. Nurse Bea offered Aubrey a Reiki session, and he gladly accepted. She said whenever she came up to visit her mother in a nearby nursing home she would stay over at L.L.'s house and come check in on us. I felt grateful. Though I could have offered him Reiki myself, I was already busier than usual with other supporting tasks.

While they were upstairs together, L.L. expressed her concerns to me. She reminded me what a big presence Aubrey had; even in his room, with his door shut, he could be a large influence, psychologically. I reminded her that I was aware of that, and had experienced living under the same roof with him, and this time seemed like a different situation than when we were married. Having him move in now felt right. And, quite frankly, it seemed to me that I was the only one in line to make such an offer.

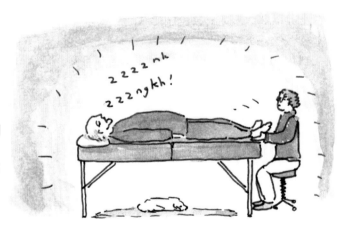

"Besides," I admitted, "I don't really think this is going to go on for very long. I don't know how long he has, but he's fading, fast. I think he's dying."

Even though I had no scientific proof for it, I sensed that it would be less than six months. A vision of helping him until mid April had flashed through my mind when I was praying, and that is what I had said yes to.

Also, I had several acquaintances who were medical professionals and healers, and when I described what I knew about Aubrey's condition, they said that this sounded like cancer in the final stage, that it was very advanced. They recommended that we get on with taking care of whatever end-of-life business there was left to do. I held this vision and informal advice in private, since Aubrey was still talking about recovery and had yet to meet with an oncologist to get a formal prognosis.

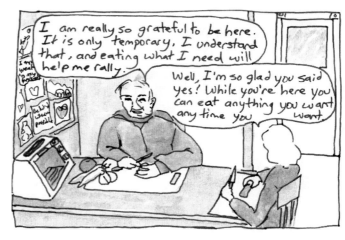

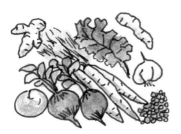

Aubrey showed me a recipe he'd found online for a juice to support healing from cancer. It seemed to contain every last ingredient one might have heard was high in antioxidants, as well as those likely to cause silent but deadly gases to be emitted from the drinker, and one ingredient that turns urine pink! Between the raw garlic and the cayenne pepper I found it bloody hard to swallow, but Aubrey's will was strong and he drank two cups of it daily as well as eating regular food.

Steve stayed and helped me around the house until late in the afternoon on Monday, January 16th, which was Martin Luther King, Jr Day, so Earl didn't have school, either. Then Steve drove home to The Big City.

On Tuesday, January 17th, Aubrey told me he had an appointment that was made weeks before with a doctor who had given him ozone therapy. This therapy had made him feel more energized, so he was looking forward to having it again. Rhia's mom, Anu, stepped up to the plate to help. Even though she had even less obligation to help than I did (they were never married), she knew I needed to drive Earl to classes and lessons, and that Aubrey was having a hard time walking, much less driving. She worked as a waitress in the evenings, so she offered to drive him to that appointment and to any future daytime appointments as well. When she arrived, she brought a rocking chair for his room and several jars of homemade soup.

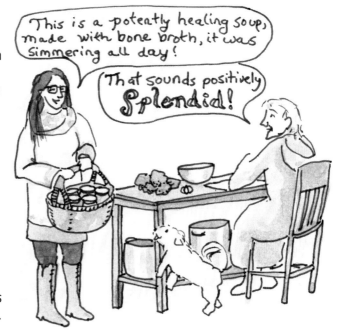

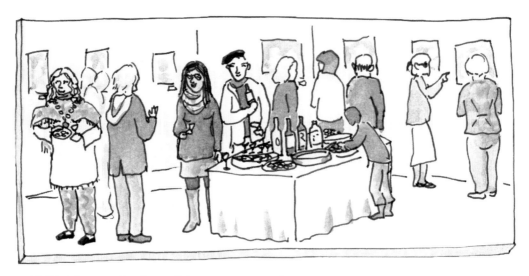

Anu and I didn't know each other well, but we appreciated each other as fellow artists. When she had time she made oil paintings of antique china and glassware, sensual photographs of vegetables and flowers, and soulful portraits. The last time we'd crossed paths was in December, at her solo exhibit. Aubrey and I had attended the opening reception (though, of course, we arrived and left in separate cars). Anu had painted a portrait of their daughter, and other characters we both knew from our community such as Moe, the founder of the Super Soup Kitchen. It is in this spirit of community that we found ourselves teaming up to help our children's father. After the ozone appointment, Anu and I discussed our concerns outside of Aubrey's hearing.

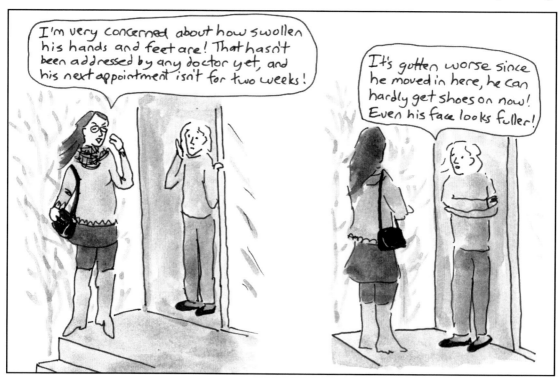

XL Baby Feet

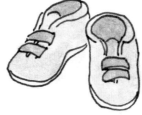

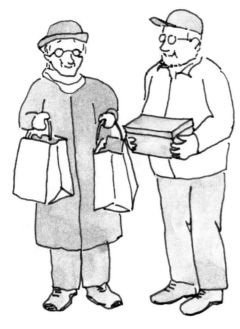

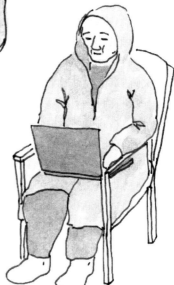

Mumsie and Grand Pops bought Aubrey new larger shoes with Velcro straps, size XXL and XXXL sweat pants, XXL T-shirts, and a voluminous gray cotton bathrobe, which he donned at once.

With all the swelling in his abdomen and limbs, he felt so much more comfortable in the new spacious clothing that he decided to have us put most of the rest of his clothing back in his car, which functioned as a mobile storage unit.

Tuesday evening, January 17th, I offered him a foot massage. His feet looked like giant pudgy baby feet. His legs were like sausages, with shiny tight skin. It was difficult to roll up his pants past his calves. He claimed to have no pain anywhere–which seemed remarkable–just some numbness in his toes.

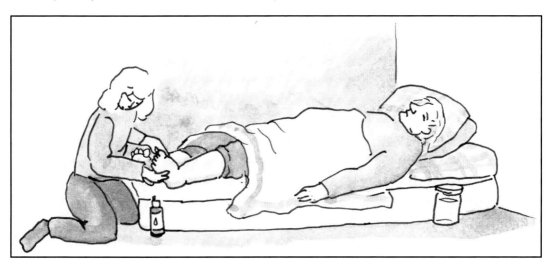

Getting the Ball Rolling

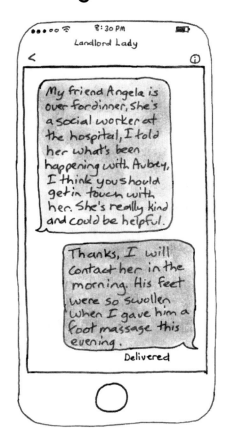

Living moment to moment, there was no bird's-eye perspective from which to appreciate the amazing choreography of what happened between Tuesday night and Wednesday morning, January 18th. Only in retrospect did the story seem to be like a ball that had been rolled, with intention, to reach a desired destination. Many details lined up perfectly:

1. Anu and I knew Aubrey much better than any doctor he had recently seen, by which to recognize the severe changes to his appearance. He was normally tall and slim, not chubby.

2. The foot massage gave further data no one else in the world had witnessed.

3. Landlord Lady happened to be personal friends with a hospital social worker named Angela, and during a casual dinner party conversation L.L. decided to mention our situation.

4. L.L. gave me contact information for Angela, whom I casually called the next morning.

5. When I explained to Angela about Aubrey's huge baby feet, she advised me to bring him to the hospital's Emergency Room, "to get the ball rolling" and "get him into the system."

Aubrey was not very interested in going, but he consented after Earl and I both urged him. We drove to the ER casually, after a late breakfast. To keep Earl on track, I asked him to work on his home-school workbooks, and I came home briefly to give him lunch and drive him to his early afternoon Social Studies class at school.

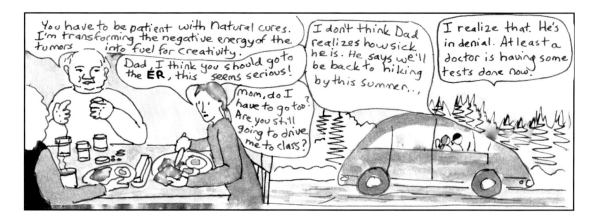

Small Brick Hospital

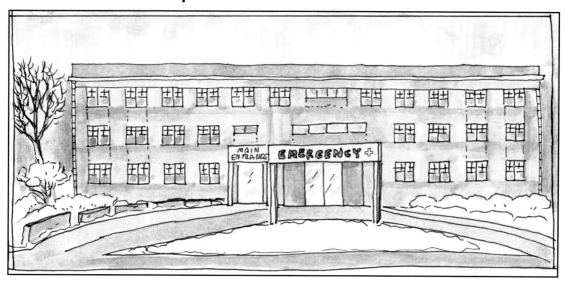

Small Brick Hospital (hereafter called SBH) was an easy dog walk from my house, and so short a drive as to make one feel self-conscious about wasting gas if one drove, unless one's passenger was hobbling, as Aubrey was. I had never been admitted myself, but Earl had, a year before, when he broke his arm. From that episode we'd gained a positive impression of the place. We'd felt respected, and conversations with doctors and nurses were as long as needed and never rushed. I appreciated the combination of living in a small, mostly rural community, with easy access to such a high-quality hospital. The fact that it was independently owned, and expertly staffed by mostly local professionals and volunteers who were one's neighbors, gave it its charm.

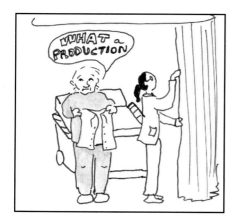

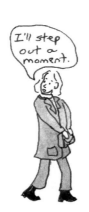

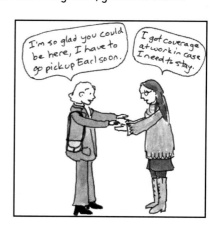

Much to Aubrey's annoyance, he was asked to put on a skimpy little robe. The ER doctor on duty ordered some exploratory tests: an ultrasound and x-rays of his torso, and an EKG. I texted Anu to let her know what was up. She said she would drive right over. When she arrived I left briefly to make Earl lunch and drive him to school. I told him of the three tests. When I got back to the hospital there was a meeting with Angela, Aubrey, Anu, myself, and the ER doctor, in which we learned what the tests had revealed.

Pressure on the Heart

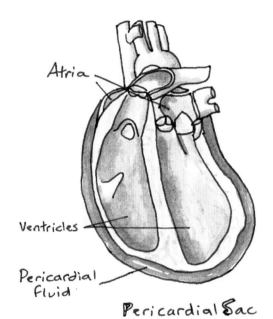

Atria

Ventricles

Pericardial Fluid

Pericardial Sac

What Aubrey described, when asked how he felt:
"I don't feel any pain, just some numbness on the soles of my feet."

What I remember a doctor, almost in tears, describe:

"as bad as I've ever seen it"
"very advanced melanoma"
"large tumors all over the torso, in many organs"
"liver failure may soon be around the corner"
"tumor in gall bladder might soon precipitate pain"
"so much fluid built up in the pericardial sac"
"the heart is under immense pressure"
"heart failure is imminent"
"surgery, a drain in the heart, could reduce pressure"
"need to be seen by a cardiologist and oncologist"
"calling an ambulance, transport to a larger hospital"

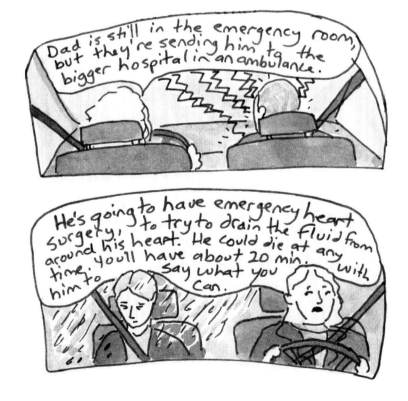

Last Words

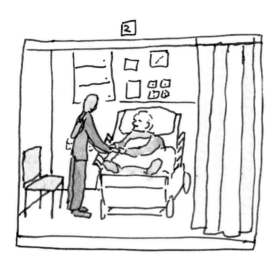
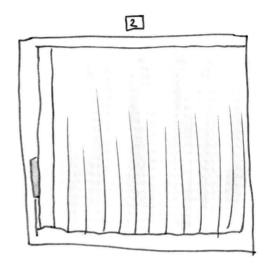

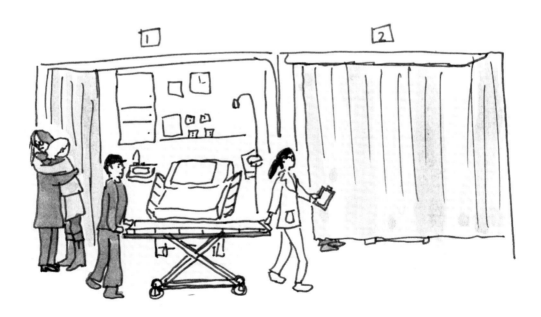

3.

Medical Interventions

New Vocabulary

In the midst of hearing doctors and nurses talking about Aubrey's tumors and heart, in the midst of taking Earl to school and picking him up and taking him to the hospital, in the midst of last minute conversations of a personal nature, I learned some new vocabulary. The hospital social worker, Angela, helped Aubrey fill out an Advance Directive and a Health Care Power of Attorney.

An Advance Directive is a written statement of a person's wishes regarding medical treatment. It is made to ensure those wishes are carried out in case that person is unable to communicate them to a doctor.

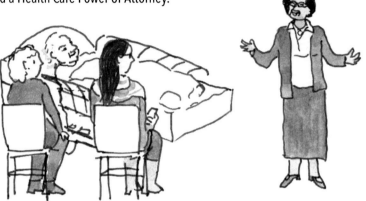

The health care power of attorney is a document in which you name someone to be your representative, or agent, in the event you are unable to make or communicate decisions about all aspects of your health care.

Anu and I decided we were most comfortable sharing the health care POA responsibilities, being teammates with equal legal status. We would also be Aubrey's health care advocates, going along with him to appointments, taking notes, supporting his wishes, and figuring out whom to talk to if he had questions or concerns. Both forms were filled out and signed by the time the ambulance was ready. Copies were made to send along with Aubrey, and Angela made copies for Anu and me.

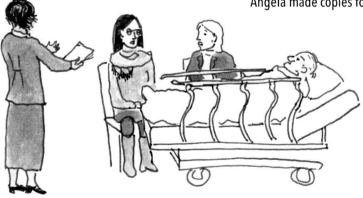

When Aubrey was wheeled away, none of us knew if we would see him again. Anu made the choice most people would find obvious: she got in her car and followed the ambulance.

Likewise Rhia, whom we had called on the phone and texted to fill her in, felt moved to drive, through two states and a winter snowstorm, all the way to the city with the big hospital, where she would arrive after midnight.

I, on the other hand, made the choice that felt right to me at the time. The winter sun was setting, and I had been at the hospital since just after breakfast. My health was not robust, and a long drive and night at the hospital would take more than I had to offer. Earl had just had the emotional roller coaster ride of his life, hearing the news and sharing "last words" in that father-son huddle. I decided we needed to pace ourselves, not make any mad dashes, by keeping our daily routine as steady and normal as possible. So we did not follow the ambulance.

We took our chances that Aubrey would survive the surgery. I explained to Earl that even if we did drive up to the big hospital, his dad might not be in any condition to visit that evening anyway. We planned to drive up the next day instead.

Before we left for home, Angela encouraged me to make haste in getting Aubrey to fill out a will, and she advised me to do the paperwork to become his financial POA. She also offered to get me a packet of papers to fill out to help Aubrey apply for our state's low income insurance program, which would help him with some medical expenses not covered by the Medicare.

She then had a kindly chat with Earl in which he discovered, and clarified, a rather significant point of misunderstanding.

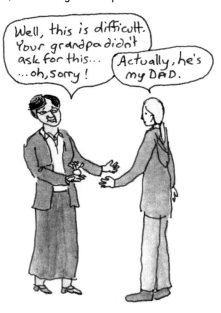

She handed him what seemed, to me, a silly little toy. (Like, "your dad might be dying, so here is this plastic flower toy, la de dah, isn't it cute?") Actually, what she said was far more sincere, and Earl received the gift with all the best intentions that it carried.

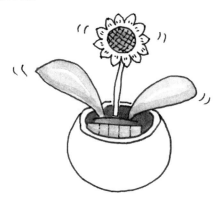

When we got home, he set it on a windowsill in the dining room next to his dad's plants. Even the tiniest level of sunlight made its solar panel work, and the little flower clicked its sincere little life-affirming dance:

"click, click, click, click, click, click"

The Big Hospital

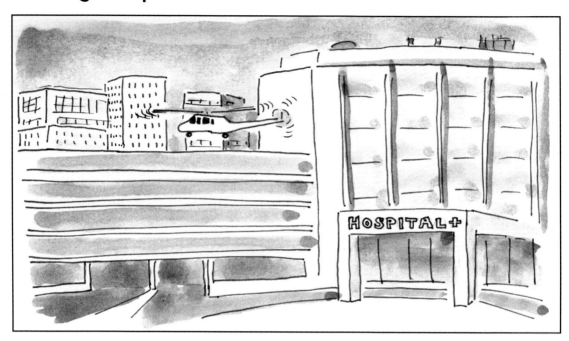

Anu texted that night to let me know that Aubrey had survived the surgery. He was in room 401, a cramped but private room in the ICU (Intensive Care Unit) in the cardiology wing of the big hospital. She stayed and spent the night in his room, not sleeping much since nurses came in every few minutes (or so it seemed) to check on him.

Rhia got there about one o'clock in the morning, Thursday, January 19th, and stayed up most of the night with her mom and dad. Then she went to the hotel near the hospital, to a room I had booked for her and Anu in case they needed it.

Meanwhile, Earl got up for his first-period Thursday French class at school. Then, back home, he tried to do a bit of his Latin workbook while I did dishes and laundry. Neither of us had the attention to focus on Algebra. We ate lunch early, and at noon began the seventy mile drive to the big hospital, aka "Modern Cement Medical Center," hereafter called MCMC.

On the way, we stopped by the Cancer Resource Center, which was largely run by volunteers and funded by donations. As Angela had promised there was a check waiting for me which covered the cost of a tank of gas and two nights at the hotel. This gesture of support warmed my heart in the midst of all the turmoil. I made a mental note to make a donation back some day.

We didn't talk much in the car. Instead, we listened to a disc of songs a friend had mixed and mailed to us. When we figured out our favorite songs we skipped over the rest and just kept cycling through those we liked. This became the theme music for the journey. Earl was the DJ. We had never been to MCMC before. As we approached it and found parking, I noted it had the impressive facade of a metropolitan airport terminal or a fancy high-rise hotel. As with an airport or a hotel, it dealt with arrivals, departures, and accommodations for its visitors, with a hefty price tag for room, board, and services.

Sibling Reunion

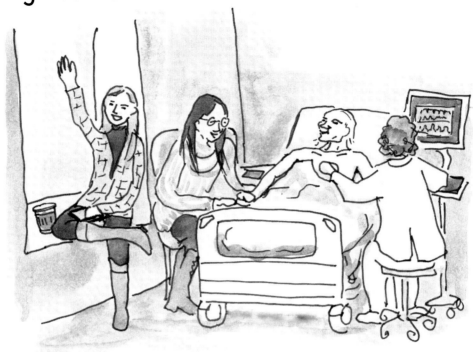

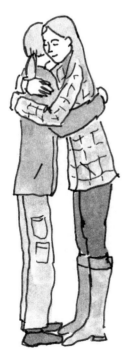

A strange, but common discovery during a health crisis is that not all of it is scary or sad. There can be unexpected moments of joy and deep love, which shine all the more brightly within that context.

In our case, the reunion of Rhia and Earl was such a moment. Being nine years apart, and never having lived under the same roof, they had not spent much time together in the past. Then, since she went away to college, and worked in another state, they had not seen one another for three years. Earl was no longer the little munchkin she remembered; now he was nearly as tall as she was!

Never mind that the place of reunion was their father's room in the ICU. Anu and I both got big grins on our faces as we watched our children embrace. As artists, who could not help but notice visual details, we couldn't help but notice how much our children resembled one another. They both had long, dark blond hair that would have been wavy if cut short. They were both tall and slender. They both had large, blue, sensitive, expressive eyes like their dad.

The man himself was able to look upon this scene and smile. His handsome chin and jawline were back to being defined, thanks to the surgery and further drainage of fluid from taking a new diuretic medication.

Being Vegan Saves a Life

Aubrey not only survived the surgery, but after having two liters of fluid drained from around his heart the first evening, and another liter drained the next morning, he felt better than he had in weeks!

None of us had realized how close to death he'd been: not weeks or days, but a few of hours at best!

Looking back, one of the little plots of our story took a positive turn. Someone I had been thinking of with annoyance, someone I had judged for being persnickety, suddenly turned out to be a heroine!

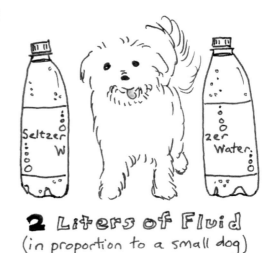

2 Liters of Fluid
(in proportion to a small dog)

How it seemed, to me, before the surgery:

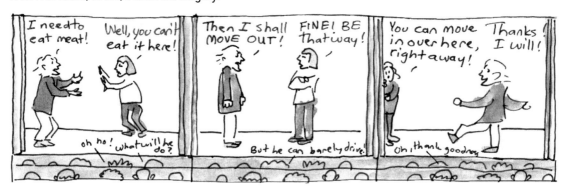

How it could have ended up, if she'd compromised:

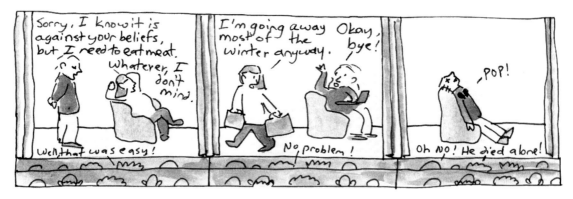

So the moral of the story is?
If you are vegan, stick to your principles! It could save a life!

Hospice?

Across the hall from Room 401, in the Family Room, Anu, Rhia, Earl, and I met with a Hospice liaison. Because Aubrey had a life threatening heart condition, as well as advanced cancer that could potentially lead to death within the next six months, he qualified for Hospice. The liaison explained that as long as Aubrey did not pursue any "curative" measures, Hospice would provide such things as a hospital bed at home, and Hospice nurses could visit our home several times a week. They could help him bathe, monitor his pain level, and help provide comfort–including administering injections of the narcotic drug morphine. The goals of Hospice care would be to assist him in feeling as comfortable as possible and to help him meet his own end-of-life goals, such as having quiet time to work on writing his book in the comfort of home. Hospice would also provide a social worker and counseling for the rest of us, to help us deal with the emotional and mental challenges that family members go through when a loved one is ill and dying.

Hospice sounded like a fine idea to me. Now that the situation had become so medically involved, I felt a bit in over my head at the idea of having Aubrey under my care all the time without anyone else looking in on him! But the choice wasn't up to me.

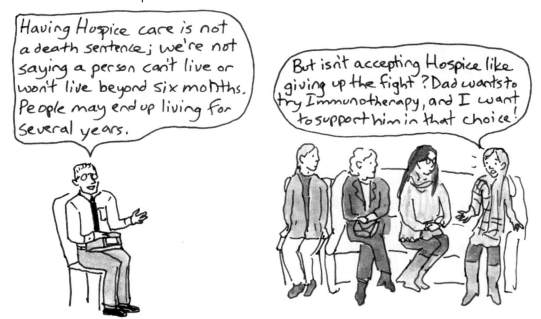

Aubrey had heard of a new form of cancer treatment called immunotherapy. It might be considered curative, or, given the advanced state of his cancer, it might only be considered palliative. No one could tell us for sure yet. If it were considered curative, he would not qualify for Hospice. Sometimes chemotherapy and radiation were accepted by Hospice if they were just for pain relief. If immunotherapy caused the tumors to stop growing or even to shrink, perhaps it could buy him some time. Perhaps it could delay the tumors in his liver causing liver failure, or the tumors in his gall bladder growing to feel like painful gall stones. He would be able to try immunotherapy if he had an MRI of his head and it showed there were no tumors in his brain. The Hospice liaison conveyed Aubrey's wish for this to the doctors, so an MRI was scheduled for later that week.

What do all those letters mean?

Here is a silly, simplistic, and by no means definitive guide to some
tests and imaging technology commonly used in modern hospitals
and some clinics. Whether you are a patient, a caregiver, or a friend
who is listening to their dramatic medical tales, it will make you feel
more savvy if you know what some of these abbreviations mean.
All of them are ways to get information about the insides of a body
without cutting it open.

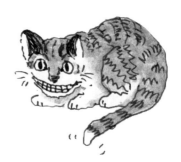

CT or CAT Scan

Obviously, this is a test where they find out if you like cats, or have cats inside you, or if you are from
Connecticut. No, not really! These acronyms refer to "Computed Tomography" and "Computed Axial
Tomography." This scan combines many cross-sectional digital X-ray images of the body using complex
math, creating 3-D images with much higher resolution (so, more information) than regular X-rays. It
can help doctors detect a variety of diseases, such as small nodules or tumors that wouldn't show up
on a plain X-ray film, and it can rapidly reveal critical information regarding conditions inside the body,
such as internal bleeding.

ECHO

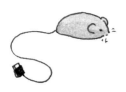

Pronounced "echo," this stands for Echocardiography and Echocardiogram.
This test is basically an ultrasound of the heart, done with sound waves
emitted by a probe that looks like a computer "mouse" which a technician
slides around on the patient's chest over some slimy sticky goo. The sound
waves bounce around inside the heart and "echo" back information, which is
portrayed as images on the screen of a monitor, showing the insides of the
heart and the blood vessels attached to it as it is pumping in real time.

EKG, ECG

Both refer to Electrocardiography. Electrodes with sticky backing are stuck onto the patient's chest,
arms, and legs. The electrodes are connected to a machine by wires. They register the heart's electrical
activity, and this is recorded and made visual as line tracings on graph paper or on a computer screen.
(This printout resembles the data shown by a seismograph, only we're studying how fast the heart is
pumping, how regular or irregular the rhythm of the heartbeats are, and the strength and timing of the
electrical impulses passing through each part of the heart, not earthquakes.) An EKG may be part of a
routine exam to screen for heart disease, stress testing, or to study heart problems such as arrhythmia,
heart attacks, and heart failure. Test results may also suggest other heart disorders.

MRI

A Magnetic Resonance Imaging scanner resembles a giant donut. The patient lies on a moving table that slides into the donut hole. This machine uses strong magnetic fields and radio waves to generate images of the anatomy, as well as to show some of the body's physiological processes. The magnetic field inside the donut is strong enough that people with some kinds of medical implants or other non-removable metal bits inside their bodies may not be able to have MRIs safely. Unlike an X-ray, an MRI can detect damage to soft tissues and nerves.

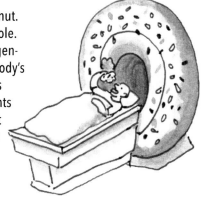

PET Scan

1. When your pet enters a room and looks around, deciding whom to rub against or lick or beg from.
2. When you take inventory of your pets to be sure they are all in for the night.
3. Positron Emission Tomography scan: The patient gets an injection of a dye that has radioactive tracers which are absorbed by the body's organs and tissues. The machine (which also looks like the donut machine above) detects the radiation and produces multidimensional colored images that show the workings of the body even at a cellular level. This can reveal a lot of information, such as if there is cancer, how far it has spread, and if a treatment has caused any changes.

Ultrasound

An ultrasound scan, also known as sonography, uses high-frequency sound waves to capture live images from the inside of the patient's body. Many people are familiar with this as a way to view a fetus during pregnancy. A hand held probe called a transducer (that mouse thing) is moved over the area being examined, sliding over a gel which helps with transmission of sound waves. This test is also used to detect some problems with organs, vessels, and tissues, and it can help guide a surgeon's movements during some medical procedures, such as when doing a biopsy.

X-Ray, Radiograph, Radiogram

When my parents were children, they could go to a shoe store and have fun putting their feet into a kind of X-ray machine, called a fluoroscope, which would show them their foot bones! Now we know that it is wise to limit our exposure to radiation and save getting zapped for when we really need it, such as to find out if we've broken a bone or need to get a wisdom tooth pulled. First, all the body parts not being X-rayed get protected by a lead-lined drape, then an electromagnetic wave of high energy and very short wavelength gets emitted by the machine. The end result is a 2D image on film. If you are lucky, they let you keep it for Show and Tell. Or, it gets digitized and viewed on a computer screen.

Going the Distance

As the sun was setting, I drove Earl back home in time for his Thursday evening fencing lesson at the YMCA, then flopped down on my bed with a massive headache. Driving 140 miles in one day was a big deal for me, much less having a family reunion and meetings about Hospice, cancer, immunotherapy, and death!

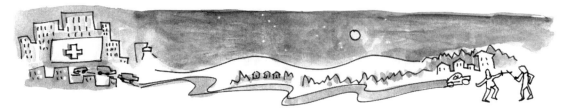

Friday morning, January 20th, Earl had French again. Then we traveled back to MCMC, listening to tunes the whole way, Earl playing DJ again. Anticipating the intensity of being at the hospital, neither of us felt moved to talk. The journey was like the pause between songs or acts in a play.

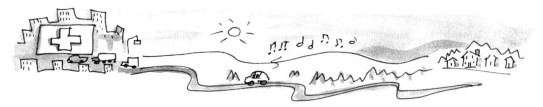

At MCMC Aubrey was sitting up in a chair! He was getting tired of being there, but wasn't yet stable enough for transport, even in an ambulance. Another half liter of fluid had been drained from around his heart. We visited for an hour and a half, then left in time to get Earl to his afternoon class at school, usually a three minute hop from our house.

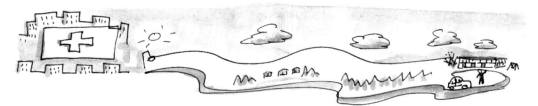

After class, my parents came over to read aloud, as they usually did on Friday afternoons. I sat with my eyes closed while listening to a chapter, then packed an overnight bag. As the sun set, I hugged them all good-bye and drove back to the city to spend the night. Earl had a sleepover at Ella's place.

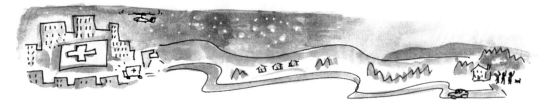

Hospital Hotel

There was a simple, old hotel very near the hospital, with low rates year round, for family members and helpers of patients. I got a room on the same floor and hallway as Anu and Rhia. Even if my reason for being there was serious, there was a certain charm to it. The old wooden desk and chair looked homey. The bathtub was scrubbed. The sink was spotless. The toilet smelled like nothing but porcelain. The bed was all made up with clean sheets. There was mood lighting as well as a bright light near the mirror, which was streak free and reflected back a rather haggard face. I lay down on the bed and stared up at the ceiling, then went to the window and peeked out. I felt secure being up in that little room with a view of the city at night: so many big buildings and vehicles, lights and shadows, and people coming and going in the parking lot down below. After eating a picnic dinner and making a weak cup of tea with the in-room coffee maker, I knocked on Anu and Rhia's door. Anu was getting ready for bed. We had a quick chat, then Rhia came to my room.

We caught up a bit: she told me about her job working with animals, and her dreams of becoming a vet. I noted that her pre-med focus had inadvertently prepared her to be able to ask very good questions when talking with her dad's doctors. This crisis was having a profound effect on her: one moment she stood in the shoes of a child, upset by the illness of her parent, the next moment she would step into a responsible adult role and ask pertinent questions which I hadn't even thought of! She also deftly took notes on her phone.

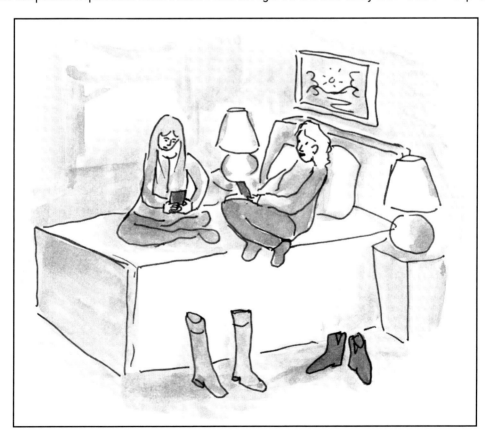

Financial Assistance

That evening, when Rhia came to my hotel room for a visit, I broached the topic of finances, and whether or not to start an online fundraiser.

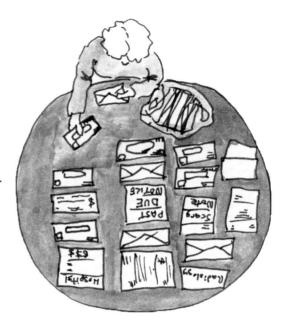

When Aubrey had filled out the application for subsidized housing, I had taken the liberty of looking over the forms to make sure he'd filled them out completely. That's how I found out that his Social Security Retirement benefit came to a "whopping" $547 per month. No one can actually retire on that amount if they live on their own! Locally, $500 could pay for a room in a shared rental house... But what about eating? And gas money? Car repairs? Dental appointments? Glasses? Printer paper? Phone? Shaving cream? Child Support?

Combine that with the fact that he had a doctor's orders, in writing, that he shouldn't drive other people (even if he could drive himself, which he could not), so he hadn't the slightest chance of returning to his former job. There were no savings or assets to be liquidated. On top of that, I found a plastic grocery bag filled with unpaid bills, going back two years. He owed Landlord Lady over $2,000, and he had outstanding medical bills from his first cancer surgery two summers before. I started to organize bills on the dining room table. But then, I had to switch to the living room floor.

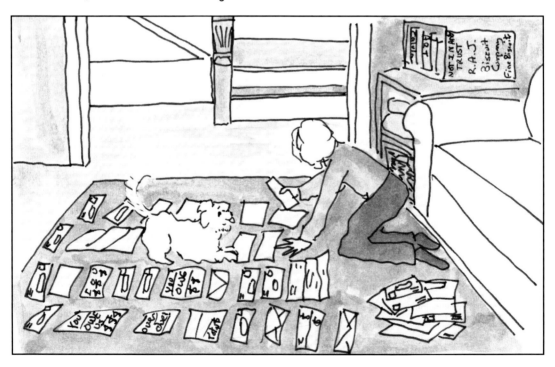

My own debts were minimal, but winter income was tenuous. While I had gotten my taxes done earlier in the month, there would be a delay until the refund, and after paying my tax guy, the credit card bill, and the utility bills for January, I had $47.00 left in the bank, no paid winter job, and no spare time to work beyond all the real-life rigamarole I had already committed to. (I spared Rhia these details.)

She was missing work to be at the hospital. Bus tickets, or gas to drive to visit her dad, cost a lot. She agreed that a fundraiser was a good idea. So, while we were both feeling brave and emboldened to ask for help, we drafted a cover story on a hotel notepad. She knew how to type faster than I did, with her thumbs, so she typed the first draft onto her phone.

As we looked through our phones' photo archives for a cover photo, we laughed together about how her dad had never liked having his picture taken. There weren't even any good ones from Christmas; he was chewing, or not smiling, or the image was blurry from us trying to snatch it quickly without him noticing.

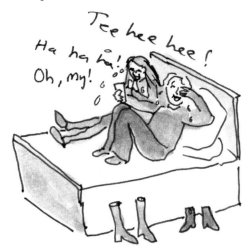

Finally, I found a photo from the previous summer. At the time, I had decided to document that familiar scene for Earl's sake, for posterity, whether or not Aubrey cared, so I'd asked them to pose for the picture.

It was a classic scene of their summer days together: Aubrey standing next to the bus he drove for the hiking camp, Earl about to join him for the hike. They would scale the mountain and return in time to meet the campers, then drive back to camp for lunch. It was the perfect image to represent him to the world!

The next decision was finding someone to help us with the confusing computer administrator part of setting up the fundraiser. I searched through my online contacts. The perfect person came to mind: This...was a job...for The TURBANATOR!

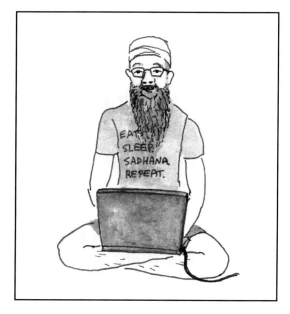

Helpful Tip: If you have to do an online fundraiser for a loved one who is dying of some terrible disease, get an account administrator who knows the patient well, who cares about your family, who is a computer geek and a good editor, who is compassionate and a good listener, so that every time you have to check in with this person to update the fundraiser goals or inform your donors of bad news, this is the person you will be dealing with.

The Turbanator fit this description perfectly! He readily agreed to help us, and by the next morning, the fundraiser was up and running!

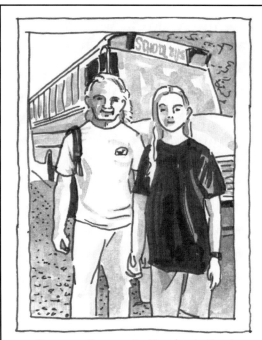

Support a Community Member in Need

~~~~

Our beloved community member Aubrey Bart is in the hospital facing life-threatening health challenges including stage 4 melanoma and a nearly fatal heart condition related to that.

He outran the grim reaper this week and intends to finish writing his opus, but has to quit his job driving buses because it is unsafe for him to drive.

His Social Security retirement benefits are not enough to live on, even as simply as Aubrey lives. There are also outstanding bills for holistic treatments that insurance wouldn't cover, dental work, car repairs, and rent.

If you would like to express your care and concern for Aubrey and are able to help ease the financial burdens associated with this condition—on Aubrey and his family—please consider making a donation today. We all thank you, and remember: what goes around comes around!

That Saturday morning, January 21st, Ella drove Earl to the hospital for a visit. It was the first time she and Rhia had seen each other in years!

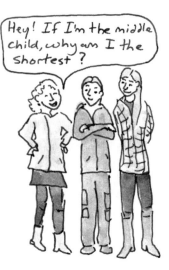

She brought Aubrey stuffed grape leaves that she'd made, one of his favorite dishes. He sat up in bed and started eating them right away, and asked about her recent travels to Athens, where she'd worked with refugees. Then he reminisced about his own youthful travels in Greece, such as the time he'd camped out in a cave by the sea! (Later, he casually added it was a good place to hide out from the cops.)

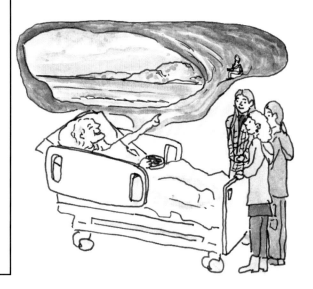

Rhia had been eating at the hospital cafeteria for days, and my breakfast at the hotel was nothing to write home about, so, for a break from the hospital atmosphere, I took Rhia, Ella, and Earl out to lunch. We found an Indian restaurant in the city.

Again, I experienced the bizarre confluence of negative events providing the excuse for some sweet sibling bonding time. Back when Aubrey and I separated the first time, just before Earl was born, I never would have imagined this scene of our three children together, having sophisticated conversations about work, travel, and politics, while eating spicy curry and rice. It brought me joy, as a mother, to watch them. And it was a treat to be eating out.

"Order a mango *lassi*, and *naan* bread too, if you want," I said, speaking from a feeling of faith in some kind of hypothetical abundance, more than certainty, "this meal is on our community."

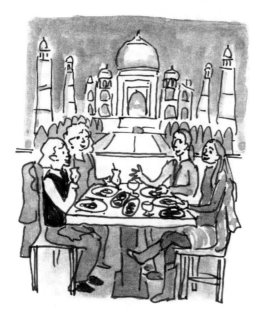

After lunch, Ella drove Earl home, and I stayed at the hospital into the evening. Landlord Lady and Nurse Bea visited. When L.L. heard about the fundraiser, and how tight money was at the moment, she wrote me a rather large check!

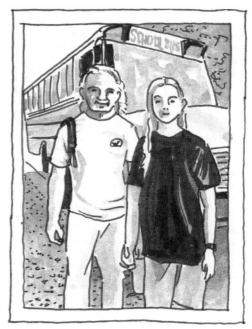

Support a Community Member in Need
~~~~
Update 1/22/17: Aubrey is still at MCMC, hoping the fibrillation in his heart can calm down enough for him to be stable enough to go home or at least be transferred to Small Brick Hospital.

Aubrey says, "Thanks for the outpouring of support. I Love Everybody."

I knew how much money Aubrey owed her for rent, and that he wanted to pay it all back, but I accepted her check, for now; it was a "cash transfussion," as Aubrey would say, to help tide us over.

My confidence that there would be community support was not misguided. But I had no idea just how much support there would be! Within the first two days of the fundraiser, Aubrey proved to have a lot more fans than I had ever imagined! As word spread through our communities, the hiking camp, in particular, people from all over the country (and beyond) made donations. Our fundraiser was given that golden word of praise: it was "trending"!

Cheers to the Bus Driver

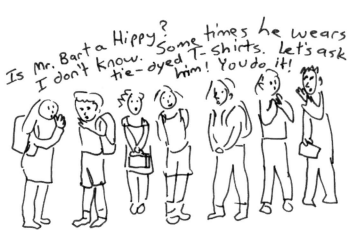

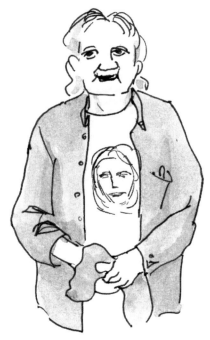

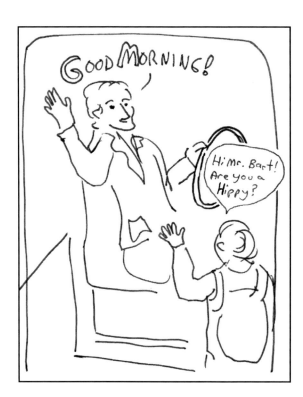

Now, it may sound ironic that a boy who hated riding the school bus, who preferred to wake up early enough to walk all the way to school, ended up becoming a bus driver. But it may be that child's aversion to bus rides which later made the man such a popular driver.

He gave everyone the time of day. He always said "good morning" as if it really were a good morning. All the students liked him, even the rascals. He had a secret place in his heart for rascals, having been one. He had an aversion to yelling and acting the role of a mean, controlling authority figure, having always disliked those himself, but sometimes he found himself having to be the person in charge when there was a wild ruckus. He'd put it to them straight, telling it like it was.

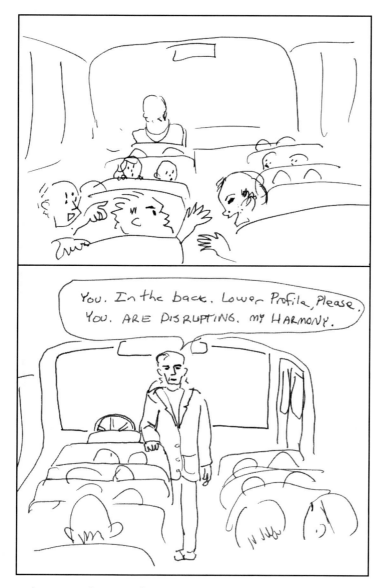

Perhaps it was his tone of voice. Perhaps it was his solemn brow. Perhaps it was shock from hearing a grown-up use such novel language. In any case, there was stone silence for the rest of that ride.

He never had any trouble from summer hiking campers; everyone on his bus was THRILLED to be there. As donations poured in online and through the mail, people also wrote comments. Here are a few:

"Even now in the middle of winter, I get a big smile thinking of getting on the bus and greeting Aubrey. Keep on truckin'." W.M.

"Aubrey has been the bus driver for the hikers for many of the close to 35 years that I have been going, and he always has a smile for everyone!" J.R.

"We so appreciate all the bus rides over the years..." P.S.

"It has been a long time since I have seen you Aubrey, but the love, kindness, and an open ear that you offered me as a little girl has never been forgotten." B.H.

"Aubrey always has such kindness for everyone." J.B.

"To a warm, simple, yet deep and extraordinary person. We love you Aubrey." C. & B.A.

"We're all concentrating on sending you positive energy and strength for your journey. Much love and gratitude for the many conversations and hikes over the years..." R.T.

"...we are so sad to hear of your difficulties. So many memories of peaceful, thoughtful, graceful times and talks with you on the school bus, on hikes...all the best, rooting for you to pull through this." D.P.

"Hello Aubrey, you're a friend of mine. Hello Aubrey, you're a friend of mine. With your hands on the wheel, we're back for every meal. Hello Aubrey, you're a friend of mine! (Loud cheering from full bus...) We love you, Aubrey!!" J.C.

Redecorating

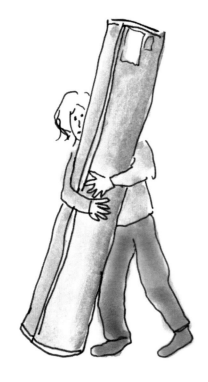

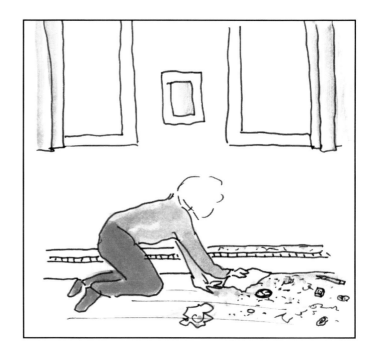

Assuming that Aubrey would need a hospital bed at home to keep his heart elevated, I spent Sunday moving the couch into the dining room, rolling up the carpet, and cleaning the floor where they had been. I also spent a long time on the phone trying to find a hospital bed to rent because, apparently, he no longer qualified for Hospice.

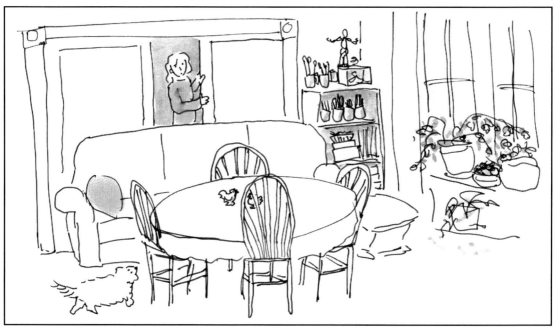

Miraculously, the MRI of his head showed that there weren't any tumors in his brain, so he got the green light to try immunotherapy as soon as he could get an appointment with his oncologist.

The next day, morning, Monday, January 23rd, I was going to go up to the hospital to relieve Anu, but she called to let me know that he was finally going to be discharged. It took hours though, waiting for various doctors to sign off that he was stable enough, and to procure his new appliance: a rolling walker. The walker was another reason to move his accommodations at home to the first floor and to take out the living room carpet. I wasn't sure how getting upstairs for bathing would work. Anu drove him home late that afternoon. She said it had been very important that she was with him at the hospital; there were so many different doctors and nurses to talk to, and it had been difficult coordinating a plan of care between the two hospitals. She was frustrated, tired, and ready to sleep in her own bed! But there were still prescriptions to be filled at the local pharmacy.

I felt a bit guilty for not having stuck it out longer at the hospital. But then again, my on-duty shift was about to begin. Leaving Aubrey alone at the house did not feel right, so Anu offered to go to the pharmacy while I helped him settle in and started making dinner. Tucker was so glad to have him back!

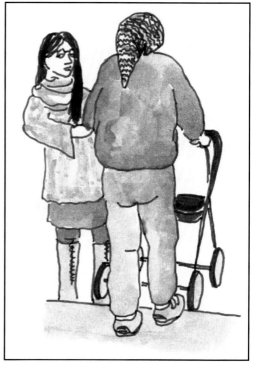

There was no bed yet, and he was very concerned about the couch being displaced into the dining room and that the living room would no longer be available for the rest of us. After he tried napping on the couch, propped up by big pillows, he proclaimed that it was good enough as a bed, so I scooted the couch back into its usual place. At least now the floor under it was clean.

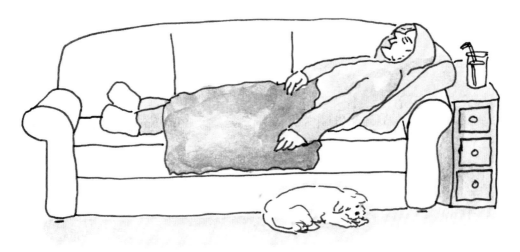

Living in the Living Room

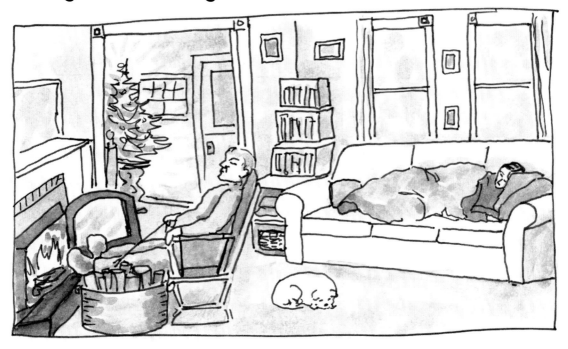

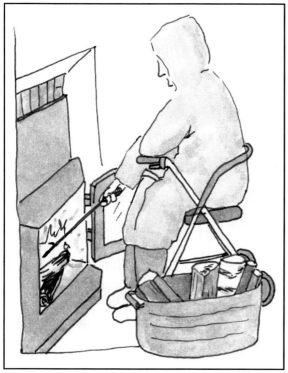

He was so glad to be out of the hospital: able to sleep whenever he wanted to, not be checked on by nurses throughout the night; able to follow his own rhythm for doing yoga, meditation, and writing; and having home cooked meals which followed his dietary interests! The dog wagged happily, and stuck close by him through dinner. Handouts from the table had been hard to come by lately.

Earl was also glad to have his dad home, though he was feeling a bit under the weather himself. One afternoon that week they napped in the living room together. The emotionally sensitive dog positioned himself exactly halfway between them.

One of Aubrey's favorite new activities was tending the fire. When I went up for bed he would still be sitting in front of the open fireplace, adjusting logs with the iron poker. We needed to keep the house much warmer than usual, for his sake.

Playing Nurse

There were new medications for him to take six times a day, a blood pressure cuff for monitoring blood pressure three times a day, and we borrowed a scale for daily weight checks. Each medicine came with pages of details. I made charts to take notes and used clipboards to keep track of everything.

He had been home for four days before we realized one important prescription had not been filled. One jar of these pills cost $364. Medicare would not cover it, and the state's insurance program had not enrolled him yet, so we had to pay out of pocket. I didn't realized that this prescription had not been filled until Angela called to tell me that she had applied for a scholarship from the hospital to pay for $300 of it. She said she would go bring that sum to the pharmacy, and I could then just pay the balance when I picked it up later. Soon she called from the pharmacy to explain that they could not accept a partial payment. So I ran out to the car, drove right over, paid the $64, picked up the prescription, and got back home within twenty minutes–the longest I felt comfortable leaving Aubrey unattended. Earl went out for a walk, not wanting to be left alone as the only first responder if anything should go wrong.

So many high stakes details! It was frightfully easy to let something important slip through the cracks! I felt like a tourist in a public park where there are rocky paths near cliffs; you could slip and break your neck, yet they allow you to hike there, unsupervised!

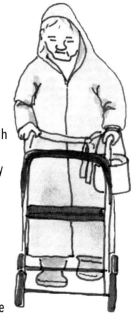

Aubrey's diuretic medication made him need to go to the bathroom at least hourly, and it was slow going with the walker through the dining room, living room, kitchen, and laundry room, to the bathroom. To compensate, he peed in a Mason jar, which he kept near the couch/bed, and then carried in a plastic bucket to the bathroom when it was full. This little pilgrimage took even more time, in order to not slosh the liquid. While I could have carried it for him, it was a chore he could still complete for himself, and the concept of him having some autonomy, taking some personal responsibility, outweighed the concept of getting the task done as fast as possible.

Part of "playing nurse," for me, was deciding when and how to back off and let him do things for himself, while still being on the lookout for when I was needed, and stepping in to help in a casual manner, so that he didn't feel like more of a burden than he already felt. He learned to take his own blood pressure, and he wrote it down along with his weight every day on the weekly chart. He took his pills on time if I left them out in a cup.

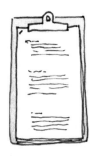
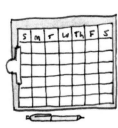
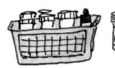

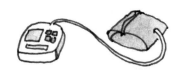

Lessons in Vulnerability

Aubrey sheepishly thanked me for helping him clean up the bathroom floor, which was hard for him to do since that involved leaning over and crouching. I told him, in all sincerity, that he had the harder role. It's much more comfortable being the one in control, on the giving end, with an identity of strength. It takes courage to admit to needing help, which can bring up feelings of humiliation and embarrassment. I spoke from personal experience.

Over the weekend, when Aubrey was still in the hospital, Moe of the Super Soup Kitchen made a spontaneous house call. He was a retired psychology professor with a buoyant personality. The soup kitchen he had founded was unusual and very popular. It was regularly patronized by doctors, lawyers, teachers, scientists, Savings & Loan CEOs, and other professionals who could afford three meals a day. The idea was to make the place a community center, staffed by volunteers, with every patron donating whatever they could afford for the hearty weekly lunches and buffet-style dinners. People came to hang out with their neighbors, hear local talent performing, and earn karmic bonus points by being of service. Aubrey always worked in the back, washing dishes. Ella was on the board, helping with publicity and fundraising. (Moe was one of her favorite people in the world.) After she got involved, I did too, painting signs and mailing thank-you cards to donors.

Moe was one of a very small group of friends to whom I'd emailed a letter explaining what was going on. Instead of just sending them a link to the fundraiser, which would have been hinting at my need as well as Aubrey's, I candidly described just how down to the last dollars I was, how little I had earned recently, that the heating bill and weekly grocery bill had gone up, and so on and so forth. I wrote to people who knew me well enough to understand how hard it was for me to share that information. Moe cut me a check for $200 to help.

(Accepting that was not the hard part.) Then he suggested doing a fundraiser dinner at the soup kitchen, during the next Family Night, coming up on the next weekend. That was harder to say yes to, but not the hardest part. We chatted a bit more. I told him about the book, *Being Mortal*, and he asked to borrow it. Then we hugged and he went on his way, most likely to his next helpful encounter.

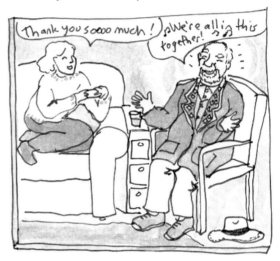

That evening, I got an email from him announcing the Fundraiser Dinner for Aubrey and Family, Saturday, January 28th. Attached to that announcement was my candid letter! When I realized that Moe had sent my personal story to over a hundred people–everyone on the soup kitchen's community and volunteer mailing list–I was mortified! I was too anxious and embarrassed to do anything besides call him up and freak out!

He explained that he had edited out a couple lines, and that my story was honest and clear. He said it would help people understand why we were doing the dinner. It answered all the questions they might have asked. Then he coached me, "This is an opportunity for you to practice feeling vulnerable, and to open up to being helped."

Bam. So. I took a deep breath, and agreed to take the psychology professor's advice.

Free Food

Somehow, I'd gotten the idea that when a person becomes critically ill or dies, then friends and neighbors deliver hot dishes and casseroles for the freezer. Perhaps my parents or grandparents had told me this, or I'd read it in a book, but I had never experienced it before, so the idea seemed weird to me. Why would the relatively healthy living members of the deceased or ill of one's family suddenly not be capable of cooking for themselves, and how would anyone know what sort of food to feed them? It took being in the shoes of the able-bodied caregiver to understand just what a balm free food could be. I was so busy preparing what Aubrey liked and needed, making our growing boy four meals a day, doing extra housekeeping and laundry, buying groceries for three, driving Earl places, making and taking phone calls, coordinating visitors, administering pills on time, and taking care of the diabetic dog, that I lost all interest in cooking or baking for pleasure. Making meals out of ingredients was pure drudgery. Following recipes was just too much.

I lost track of my own appetite when looking into the refrigerator full of herbal supplements, beet juice, bone broth, and cold raw vegetables. So, when I was offered the opportunity to receive five free meals a week, for the three of us, from a local volunteer organization that helped families who were afflicted by cancer, I was ready to say yes, no matter what kind of food was delivered! When a volunteer named Aladdin showed up on the front porch with the bags, it was like a happy dream: broccoli quiche and shepherd's pie, how comforting! Seafood linguine and roasted Brussels sprouts with red grapes, how exotic! It was nothing I would have made the effort to prepare for myself, and it sparked my appetite. I felt more secure, and cared for, in a deep primal way.

To make the situation even better, Aladdin was a cancer survivor himself, and he knew how to give kind counsel to families in need. He reached out to Earl as a big brother would, inviting him to hang out some time, talk about his dad, or just have a fun outing to get away from the house. What more could a mother have wished for?

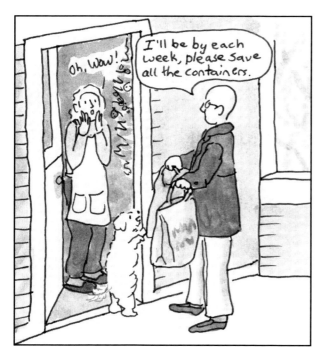

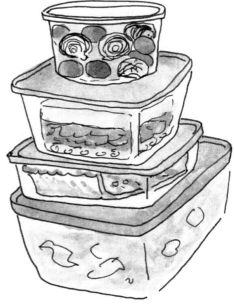

Expeditions and Adjustments

Now that his dad was no longer taking walks, Earl had to decide if he was going to stay inside all day, accept me as an alternate walking partner, or venture out by himself. He tried the first for a while. Winter weather and school made valid excuses. He tried the second, but concluded that I talked too much.

Finally, he felt enough cabin fever to venture out on his own, and found it enjoyable enough to do frequently. It was heartening to hear him say, "I'm going out for a walk, Mom," and know that he would find some solace in nature—and that he didn't require his dad's presence to access this. Also, it was clearly a shift into a more independent phase of his life.

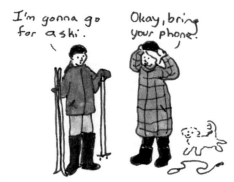

He could have taken Tucker, but picking up dog poo was not on his agenda. The old dog was only up for short walks, anyway, and Earl, alone, was often out for more than an hour.

So, all the dog walking fell to me. Often I felt too tired to have a strong opinion about which direction to go, so I let Tucker lead. He would usually walk us up the street to the library, where the nice librarian ladies would give him biscuits!

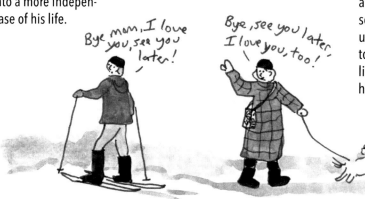

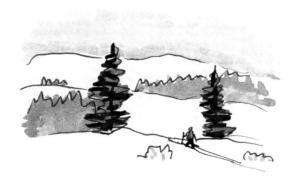

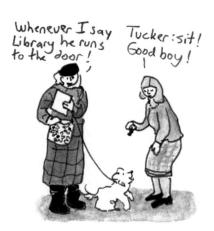

In spite of the serious medical reasons for our physical proximity, this unlikely period of shared residence with my ex-husband had its warmth and sweetness. Freed of the expectations of marital partnership, we were able to appreciate one another's company. He worked on his book, slept, and took care of his body as best he could. I focused on basic maintenance of the house, dog, boy, and whatever Aubrey needed help in doing. A tentative hug and "Good night, I love you," turned into a routine we both observed and never discussed.

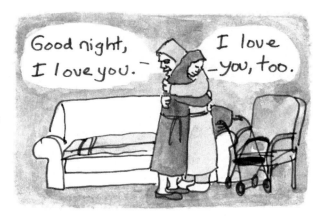

Earl preferred to practice music while his dad was out of the living room. Sometimes a long bathroom break or being out for a doctor appointment provided this window of opportunity. I cherished hearing the music, including the warm-up scales, missed notes, and repeats; it gave life to the atmosphere of the house, and represented incremental progress.

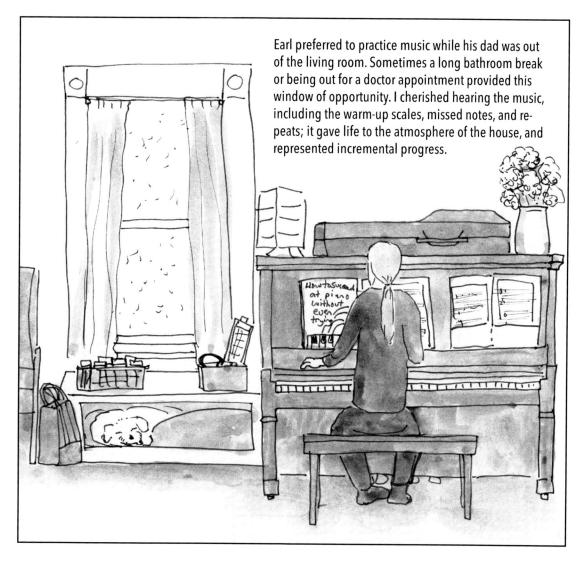

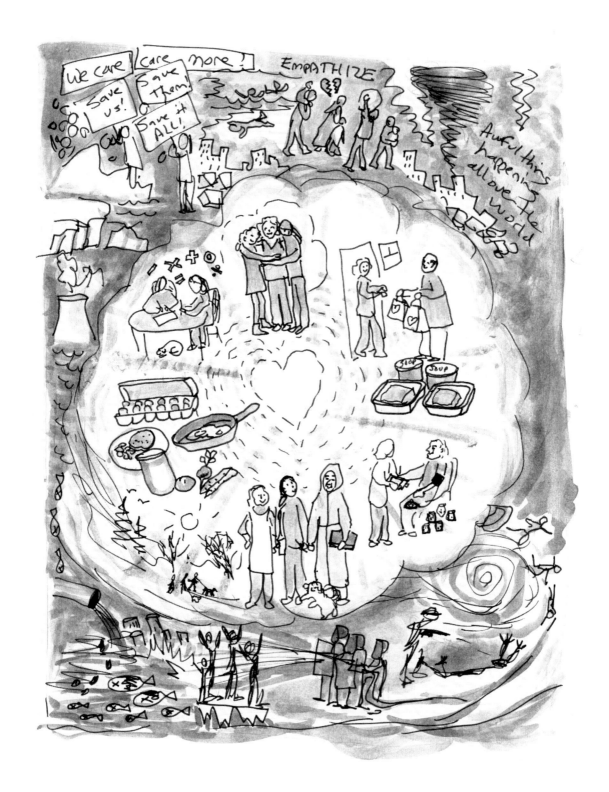

Before Aubrey moved in, I often checked various online news sources to keep tabs on the headlines. In general, this precipitated feelings of angst. Facebook, the virtual meeting place where I carried out most of my friendships, was the most unnerving. Scrolling down through the posts, scanning text and images, one never knew what one might encounter: a friend's cute toddler, or a plea to help save a child from famine; beauty or violence, celebration or outrage. Should one try to stay mentally detached, or tune in but risk emotional whiplash? As my therapist said in our monthly visits, scanning Facebook was "highly dysregulating." Still, it was my primary portal for communication with friends and community far and near.

After Aubrey moved in, I waited a while to see how it was going before sharing any posts about it. When I reflected on those ten days, I realized that in spite of how much work it was, the overall tone of daily life had changed in a surprising way: in the face of all the world's problems, I felt buffered! There was freedom in no longer wondering what causes to join; I felt permission to not worry about all the rest because I was already doing the most that I could do to help. I wasn't in charge, and there was no plan beyond the daily routines, so it was easier to live in the moment. There was a glow of grace permeating everything, and a calmness, as if I were resting in the eye of a hurricane.

Facebook post Tuesday, January 24:

I've got it all. I really do: Two amazingly resilient children, even when one is not feeling well she manages to bring more light into the room and a warm comfort to her brother, who is going through some of the most challenging times a child can go through, witnessing the illness of a parent, yet he keeps a sense of humor and an even keel, and helps with chores and cares about keeping up in school, and goes deep into contemplation about existential questions; an adoring boyfriend who recognizes what I'm going through with family health crises and who offers to clean bathrooms when he visits, who supports all my choices and helps me laugh and listens to me whine and reassures me that I can be as involved as I need to be and he thinks I am doing the right thing; an opportunity to keep loving an ex-husband who is now a dear friend and has always been a dedicated dad to our son, going for a walk or hike almost every day of our son's life until recently, a man who is now humble and wise enough to recognize he needs some help and to allow for it to be given—I love seeing him wearing his new hooded monk's robe, feeding the fire, being able to hug and smile and eat chocolate together—I'm learning to take blood pressure and make pill charts and fill out legal paper work—we are pulling together to get this work done—and on the team is the mother of his daughter, and they are both phenomenal women, with great big hearts, part of the intelligent caring team of support, showing up after an all night drive from out of state, showing up for early morning pick-ups to go to appointments, showing up to stay overnight in the hospital, asking excellent questions and taking notes, helping in every way they can; and another ex-husband, dedicated father of our daughter, who is open minded and big hearted enough to embrace the other one.

I perceive a sense of continuity coming into focus; rather than a timeline broken into fragments labeled with one relationship or another, I'm seeing and feeling what holds it all together, and I get to love them all, and it is so good to not need to hold anything back anymore.

Financial POA

Tuesday, January 24th, I went to the local bank to take care of more legal paperwork that Angela had recommended.

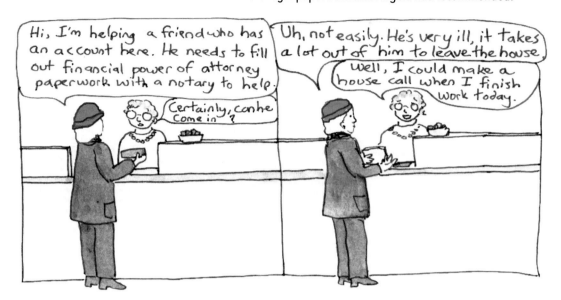

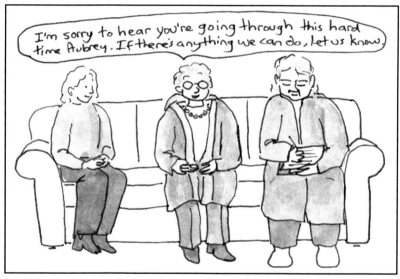

After the notary's kind house call, I had legal permission to see all of Aubrey's checking account transactions, keep track of the balance, and write checks from his account–as long as he was alive.

I also gave his account number to The Turbanator, who gave it to the online fundraiser, so that the first wave of donations could be transferred.

There were so many bills to pay that I wasn't logically certain where to begin. So I applied a tactic that had been helping me figure out what to do in other areas of life when I felt overwhelmed: in my imagination, I handed all the money over to an invisible holy higher power, and asked for guidance about what to do. The next day, while driving, not thinking about money, all of a sudden I got a vision of several checks being written, to whom, and for how much. This seemed so clear that I laughed out loud. When I shared this vision with Aubrey, he accepted it and wrote the checks without question. Some people might think this was crazy, but for the two of us this was not unusual. In fact, one of the ways we had always been compatible was our comfort with and acceptance of this way of navigating in life that went beyond rational understanding.

Brothers

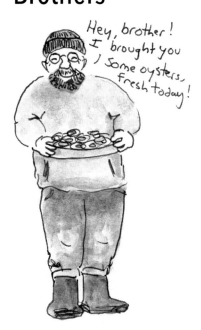

Wednesday, January 25th, Aubrey and I got up very early so as to be ready when Anu came at 7:00 a.m. to drive him to a cancer care center in the city near MCMC. He was getting a PET scan. Earl and I did school that morning. When they came back, Anu needed to leave for work, but Earl and I had our own medical appointments to go to, so two of Aubrey's friends took turns hanging out with him. The Farmer brought one of Aubrey's favorite treats: fresh oysters! The Turbanator taught yoga classes up at the college, which Aubrey used to attend, so while they were visiting they did some gentle stretches and breathing exercises together.

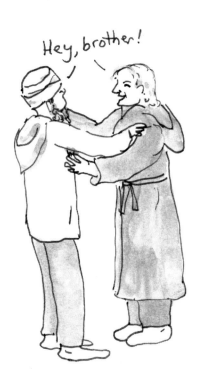

Soon after Earl and I got home and these friends had gone, there was a knock at the door: it was Aubrey's brother and sister-in-law! Mark and Betty had been driving for two days–ever since they found out about the cancer. Their daughter, friends with Rhia, had read about it on Facebook! Certainly not the best way to find out! That was one of the biggest balls that had been dropped. Fortunately, no time was wasted with hurt feelings. The brothers got right down to business reminiscing about their youth, which was very amusing!

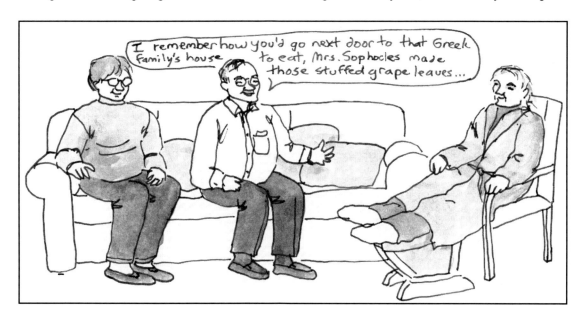

Tales of Wild Bill

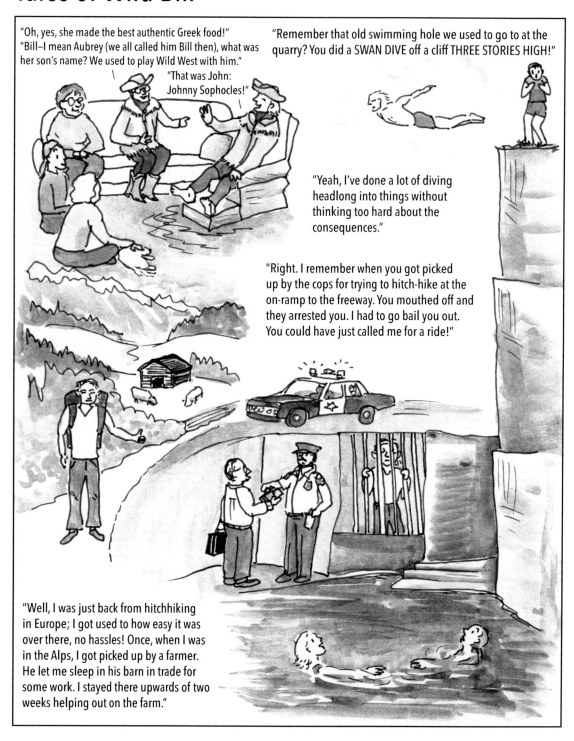

"Oh, yes, she made the best authentic Greek food!"
"Bill—I mean Aubrey (we all called him Bill then), what was her son's name? We used to play Wild West with him."

"That was John: Johnny Sophocles!"

"Remember that old swimming hole we used to go to at the quarry? You did a SWAN DIVE off a cliff THREE STORIES HIGH!"

"Yeah, I've done a lot of diving headlong into things without thinking too hard about the consequences."

"Right. I remember when you got picked up by the cops for trying to hitch-hike at the on-ramp to the freeway. You mouthed off and they arrested you. I had to go bail you out. You could have just called me for a ride!"

"Well, I was just back from hitchhiking in Europe; I got used to how easy it was over there, no hassles! Once, when I was in the Alps, I got picked up by a farmer. He let me sleep in his barn in trade for some work. I stayed there upwards of two weeks helping out on the farm."

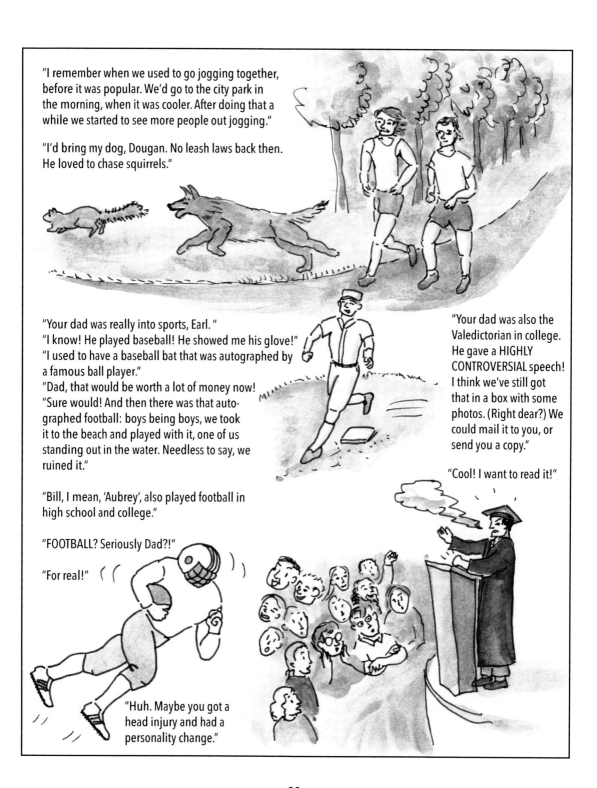

"I remember when we used to go jogging together, before it was popular. We'd go to the city park in the morning, when it was cooler. After doing that a while we started to see more people out jogging."

"I'd bring my dog, Dougan. No leash laws back then. He loved to chase squirrels."

"Your dad was really into sports, Earl. "
"I know! He played baseball! He showed me his glove!"
"I used to have a baseball bat that was autographed by a famous ball player."
"Dad, that would be worth a lot of money now!
"Sure would! And then there was that auto- graphed football: boys being boys, we took it to the beach and played with it, one of us standing out in the water. Needless to say, we ruined it."

"Bill, I mean, 'Aubrey', also played football in high school and college."

"FOOTBALL? Seriously Dad?!"

"For real!"

"Huh. Maybe you got a head injury and had a personality change."

"Your dad was also the Valedictorian in college. He gave a HIGHLY CONTROVERSIAL speech! I think we've still got that in a box with some photos. (Right dear?) We could mail it to you, or send you a copy."

"Cool! I want to read it!"

New Aunt & Uncle

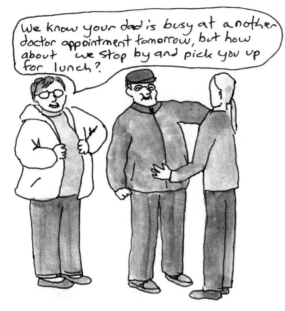

We know your dad is busy at another doctor appointment tomorrow, but how about we stop by and pick you up for lunch?

Once again, the health crisis was a catalyst for an unexpected good thing: For Earl, it was a bonus to have a brand new aunt and uncle! He found it fascinating to hear his uncle's version–the younger brother's perspective–of stories his dad had told him.

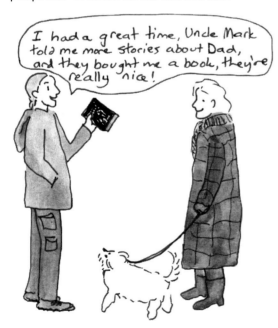

I had a great time, Uncle Mark told me more stories about Dad, and they bought me a book, they're really nice!

How is it possible that they had never met before?

Aubrey had always dreamed of taking Earl on a road trip. He loved a good road trip. Called himself a "Road Scholar" even. Before Earl was born, Aubrey used to visit his brother's family on his annual pilgrimage to the Jazz Festival in New Orleans. That's how his niece got quite fond of her somewhat eccentric and free-spirited uncle. When Rhia was little, Aubrey took her to meet them, and later she visited them on her own. But for most of Earl's childhood, his dad had driven buses year round, even double shifts through the summer months. Earl was either too young to travel, or there wasn't enough time or money to get away for a journey together.

Having finally been introduced (if under solemn circumstances), there was mutual enthusiasm on all sides to continue the relationship. They invited Earl to visit them in the summer, and offered to buy him a plane ticket. He said he'd consider it.

They stayed at an inn, close to our house, for two nights. Anu and I met with them there so we could discuss everything candidly. Naturally, they had a lot of questions! When they had last seen Aubrey, at a family wedding, no one guessed he had cancer and would have surgery later that summer! Nor did he volunteer that information after the fact. It was a shock to all of us to find out now, when the cancer was so advanced. But since there was no cure and the cancer had already metastasized, perhaps his silence had been a gift to all of us. His decision to keep it to himself seemed brave, and he'd saved us from a year and a half of worrying and feeling anguish about not being able to help him recover.

On the other hand, perhaps if he hadn't been so stoic there were things we could have done to help him live out some of his remaining dreams instead of working himself to the bone. Oh well, no use torturing ourselves with "would of, could of, should of."

Now that Aubrey suddenly needed help, Mark and Betty said they would have been open to taking him home with them, but they could see that it was important for him to stay with us, in his community, where he could have as much time as possible with his children. (Though Rhia lived out of state, it was closer to drive here, and her mom was here as well.)

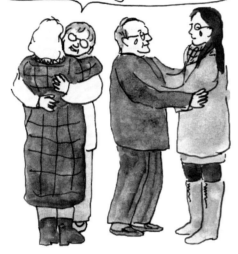

We're very sad and upset about the cancer, but we can tell Aubrey is trying to be strong and brave, and you two are certainly taking great care of him!

We were lucky to all be in agreement about this. It is common for family members to have differing opinions and beliefs when it comes to decisions about where the ill or dying person should live, who the caretakers will be, what kind of treatments should or shouldn't be used, and so on. No one is in charge of how the illness will progress or when death will come, but many people try to cope by grasping for things to control and fervently trying to make things go as they think they ought to go. Those struggles can add a level of complexity and emotional drama to a situation that is already precarious because of the loved one's failing health. An extra dose of patience and respect can help. The idea, "This isn't about you, it's what the patient needs and wants," can help guide some discussions.

Let's pretend it *is* all about you!

If you were the patient:

- What kinds of treatment and support would you value and wish to receive? (Traditional western medicine, alternative medicine, spiritual support, cutting-edge experimental treatments, everything possible, nothing at all, thank you?)
- Are these treatments and kinds of support available near you? If not, how far are you willing and able to travel to get the treatment and support in which you believe?
- Can you afford that care? If not, is there a way to change that?
- Who would you trust and reach out to for various kinds of help: emotional support, financial support, help with chores, childcare, helping you bathe, driving you places, going to appointments with you, *et cetera*.
- When ill, do you prefer privacy and solitude, or is companionship more comforting? Would you prefer quietness, or to talk, visit with loved ones, listen to music, watch TV?
- What brings you comfort? (Certain foods, music, movies, books, friends? A spiritual practice or community? Pets? Massage?)

If you were a caregiver:

- What are ways you might help someone in need? (Are you a good cook? Willing to drive to appointments? Able to watch children or tend pets? Too busy to volunteer but able to make financial contributions? Enjoy reading aloud, singing, playing guitar at bedside? Good at organizing other volunteers to cook/clean/visit?)
- What kinds of treatment and support do you value and believe are important? How might you react if the patient did not share those beliefs?
- What helps you keep yourself strong so that you don't burn out? What can you do to nurture yourself? Who can you go to for emotional support when you're frustrated, frightened, or sad?

Communication Complications

Thursday, January 26th, Nurse Bea came over and gave Aubrey a Reiki session. Then Anu came over and drove him to MCMC for an appointment as an out patient. He was having an Echocardiogram to see how his heart was doing. It had been four days since he'd been discharged from MCMC, and I had a problem to solve.

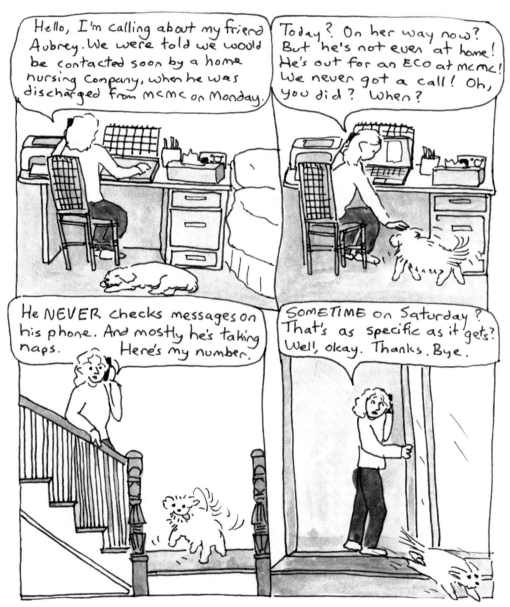

I also put in a request for a urinal, to make peeing in the living room easier and more sanitary. Whoever I talked with had access to Aubrey's chart. She must be the person who discovered that the $364 prescription hadn't been filled, because soon after this call I met Angela at the pharmacy with that balance of $64.00.

On Friday morning, January 27th, Betty and Mark stopped in to say good-bye on their way out of town. We exchanged addresses and phone numbers. I promised to keep them in the loop going forward, instead of leaving them to wait for Aubrey to tell them anything.

Then Anu arrived to take Aubrey to yet another doctor appointment. This time, thank goodness, it was at a clinic right in town, to establish new patient status with a new primary care provider, Dr. Kay. This doctor explained that one of the recent scans showed a tumor the size of a golf ball impacting Aubrey's heart, and she explained that immunotherapy would be palliative, at best, not curative. So Aubrey *did* qualify for Hospice home care services, after all!

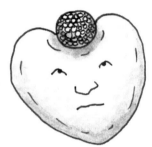

When Rhia heard about this, over the phone, she was very concerned that signing her dad up for Hospice meant we were all giving up the fight for his life. She again advocated for giving immunotherapy a chance and holding onto hope. By living so far away, she was not able to participate as much as she yearned to, nor experience all the detailed conversations by which to sense and trust that there was a supportive atmosphere. She was aware of that disadvantage, and was starting to seriously considering quitting her job and moving back home. We all felt the challenge of not knowing how long any of this would go on.

Saturday, January 28th was as busy as the rest of the week had been. I had an appointment for which I needed coverage. Several community members had offered to help, in theory, but when it came to pinning down a specific person to cover a specific time, the project felt like solving an SAT question. Lining up a sitter took until the last minute.

The concept of "asking for help" *sounds* reasonable, but it was not so easy to delegate the most stressful and demanding tasks. What took the most time and attention were not things I could hand off to anyone else, such as waiting for call backs, filling out paperwork, and making business related phone calls. With pills, meals, and cleaning up messes, there was a feeling of needing to be constantly "on call." Sometimes when I thought I had coverage, or someone had offered some kind of help, someone forgot and I had to search for a substitute.

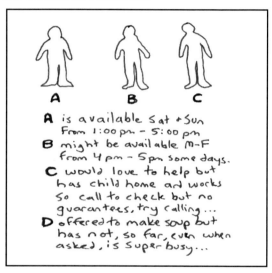

That Saturday, as soon as I came home through the back door, there was a knock at the front door. A kindly and sensible looking stranger turned out to be the visiting nurse! Finally! I was certainly glad I hadn't missed her! She explained why they couldn't plan specific times for visits: there were so many patients on the list, and each visit would take however long it would take. I had hoped she would bring a urinal, but my request had not been passed along to her. The purpose of her house call was to explain about the program and to establish contact. Some other new nurse would be assigned to Aubrey and visit us the following week. When I brought up his doctor's statement that he qualified for Hospice, she was surprised. This effectively canceled Aubrey's need for the home care program she represented!

Of Wills and Will Power

Aubrey wasn't so sure that he wanted to be signed up for Hospice, anyway. In spite of attempts by me and others to explain the benefits (for other family members as well as himself) he still saw accepting Hospice care as "giving up."

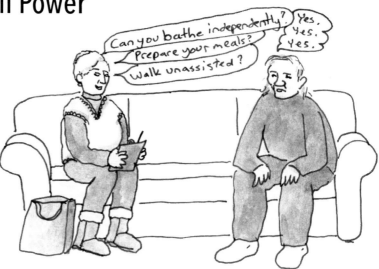

As the visiting nurse questioned him about his current abilities, his responses belied a different perspective than I held, and I felt frustrated.

Just the day before, while talking with Angela about the pharmacy, I had to ask her for a new copy of a disability application. On the old form, Aubrey had significantly overestimated his abilities and independence, so the form needed to be redone for him to qualify. When I picked up the fresh form at SBH, Angela wrote CANCER at the top, and underlined it, so as to expedite the processing, which usually took weeks. Then I went home and filled it out again, and simply had Aubrey sign it.

Angela had also been coaching me to help Aubrey fill out a will as soon as possible. To Aubrey, making a will was a sign that I was planning for his death rather than being positive and hoping for the best. He didn't see himself as being near the end. I tried to explain that many people make out their wills much earlier in life, long before they suspect the end may be near, and then edit them as times goes by. When he finally agreed, making a basic will was fairly quick and easy, as he had no real estate, no stocks or bonds, no life insurance, and no bank account savings other than the online donations, which we were using to pay off his back rent and other old unpaid bills, and to buy things he needed right away, such as the rolling walker and the fancy pills.

State insurance might have covered the latter two, but it still hadn't been granted. (Medicare would only pay 80% of expenses outside of the hospital, leaving a 20% co-pay for the ill, disabled, and unemployed patient to magically provide.)

Dealing with forms was frustrating, but my biggest challenge, in terms of Aubrey's take on his situation, was running interference between him and pretty much everyone else! Most people, upon hearing about stage 4 melanoma, a body riddled with tumors, and a heart on the verge of failing, assumed that death was on its way, sooner than later. I had to brace myself for their responses, remembering that I was used to the news but for them it was freshly devastating.

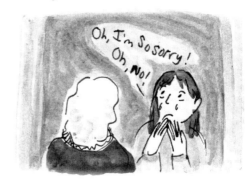

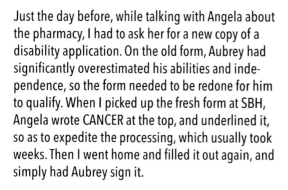

Perhaps death could be stalled through immuno-therapy, but the adage, "hope for the best while preparing for the worst," seemed practical to me. In other words, it might be a good idea to let people far away know, so they could have the chance for one more visit. Allowing friends and family the chance to reminisce, as his brother had, in case this was near the end of their earth-walk together, could provide some closure for everyone.

But Aubrey was not interested or ready to entertain such thinking. He didn't want me to try to contact any of his old friends. The story he told himself—and anyone who would listen—was that cancer was only a temporary setback. He was aiming to completely overcome the disease through immunotherapy, meditation, prayer, positive intentions, herbal sup-plements, and special diets. His expressed hope was to be back on the hiking trails by summer.

Of course, no one wanted to crush his spirit and take away his hope, so we all listened and nodded and smiled. (His optimism was certainly easier to witness than if he had acted sad, angry, or depressed.)

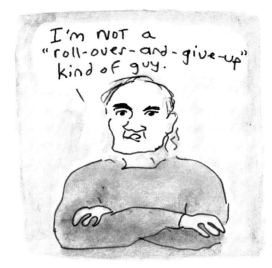

He was so optimistic that if people called him and asked to visit they might not understand just how advanced the cancer was, so they wouldn't be prepared for how different he looked, sounded, and smelled. For their sake, I tried to prepare them (at least a little), by describing some of what I was witnessing at home and then coaching them. "He's really not interested in discussing death and dying, or having 'closure' type of conversations. He doesn't see this as the beginning of the end, and he may simply stop responding and ignore you if you start saying things to that effect."

My coaching seemed like spin control, but I also felt it was part of "holding the space" for his process. Perhaps this was truly helpful, or perhaps it was a dysfunctional pattern left over from our marriage, of me trying to hold open a space for him which wasn't necessary, nor my job to hold.

Who knows? Sometimes there isn't an obvious "right answer;" we're all just winging it.

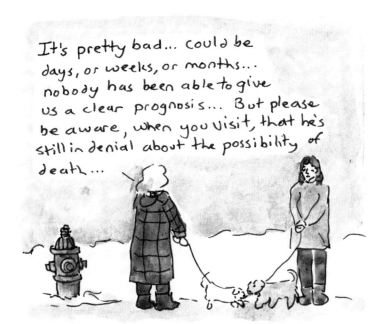

Fundraiser Supper

Saturday evening, January 28th, while friends stayed with Aubrey, Earl and I got up our nerve to go to the Super Soup Kitchen supper that Moe had publicized. Steve was up for the weekend, so that gave me some comfort. I was nervous about being in the spotlight, asking for money, and was not sure who would be there or how many people would come out on a cold winter's night. Moe's eyes twinkled as he gave me a big hug. As the dining hall filled up, it was apparent that Aubrey had a lot more local fans than I'd imagined! Most people who dined that night knew him as their bus driver, or as their children's driver, or both! As for feeling vulnerable, few people even knew who Earl and I were, so we were able to relax and melt into the crowd and enjoy the delicious food and live music. Others took care of everything. That was such an amazing gift!

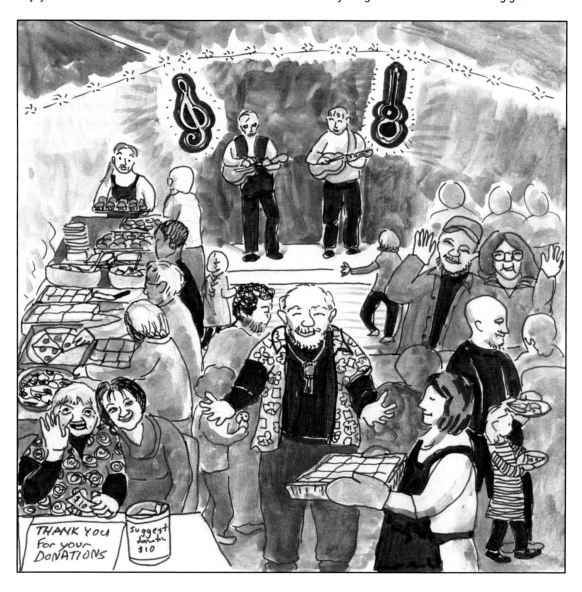

Facebook post Sunday, January 29:

Thank you to everyone at the soup kitchen for last night's awesome fundraiser for Aubrey! Great classic Beatles music by the band! We are all feeling so blessed to live in such a supportive community. I didn't know many people, but it is clear that Aubrey has many friends, from bus driving for the elementary school routes, the high school, the town, and for the hiking camp. Thanks to everyone who helped spread the word!

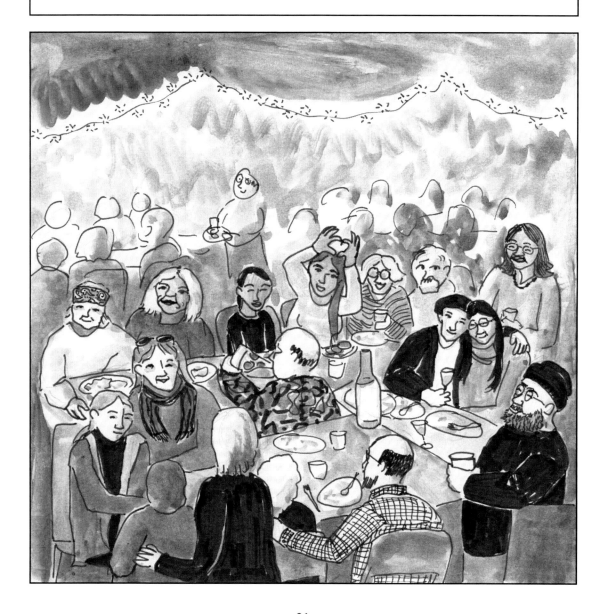

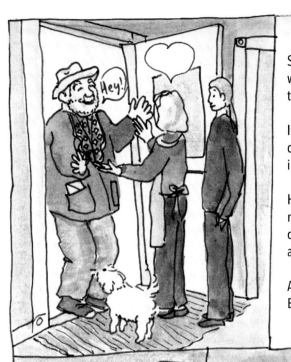

Soon after the fundraiser supper, while Earl and I were struggling to do a bit of home-school math, there was a knock on the front door. A reprieve!

It was Moe, with an envelope stuffed full of cash donations! We had never beheld so much money in cash before! $1,138.00, to be precise!

He couldn't stay long, so we gave each other merry hugs and I thanked him for everything he'd done to help us. He reminded me that what goes around comes around.

After we said good-bye and he drove out of sight, Earl had the best math class ever!

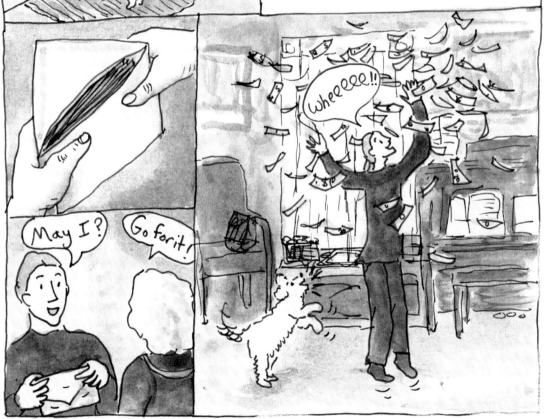

Partying and Praying

With Aubrey living in my house, the living room became a multipurpose meeting hall for family, friends, visitors from away, visiting nurses, and on Sunday, January 29th, a prayer and sacred song meeting called "Kirtan." Although I was glad to play hostess to whatever was necessary and helpful, I didn't feel interested to join the group that was planning to gather for Aubrey's sake that night, so when this event was organized, I supported it by vacuuming the floor and lighting a bunch of votive candles. As soon as Anu, Rhia, and others began to arrive, Steve, Earl, and I went to Ella's dad's house for a Chinese New Year themed dinner party.

At the party everyone was wearing something red for good luck, and we all helped to make steamed buns, filled with vegetables, pork, mushrooms, and sweet red bean paste. They were delicious! It felt very refreshing to have a whole evening that had nothing to do with caregiving, cancer, medical procedures, or administrative paperwork! The only sad part was Steve needing to leave part way through to drive home to The Big City. At least it was a calm, clear, starry night, good for driving.

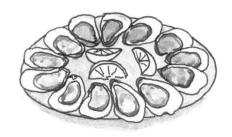

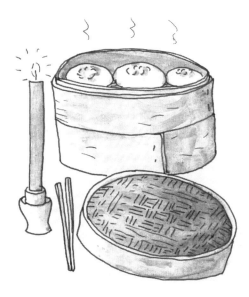

When Earl and I returned to our house, Aubrey was enjoying some raw oysters that The Farmer had brought him. A fire was glowing in the fireplace, and the room was still softly lit by candles. Around the room there were photocopied pages of prayers, written phonetically and in mysterious Sanskrit letters, which everyone who came must have chanted. The sacred meditation, "Ra Ma Da Sa," was for sending prayers of healing to a loved one.

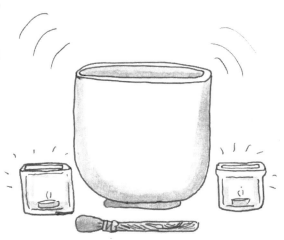

There was a new *objet d'arte* in the living room, a tall white crystalline bowl which toned a long beautiful note when hit with a mallet. Apparently this tone supports the heart specifically. The Farmer said we could hang onto it for the time being.

Anu said the gathering had been beautiful. Before she headed home, we firmed up plans for the next day: she would come at 5:00 a.m. to take Aubrey to yet another ECHO at the cancer care center. I would have his charts and meds packed to go along.

The Pressure Continues

Monday, January 30th, there were still stars in the dark winter sky when we arose. So far, we'd been lucky to have good weather for all these long drives and appointments, no icy rain or snow storms, not even any treacherous blowing and drifting snow. Anu pulled up on time, and I was so glad she was taking on this chore. After handing her the bag with all the medicine bottles, and the clipboard with the week's data on weight, blood pressure, and pills, and helping Aubrey on with his coat, I took the liberty of going back to bed.

A few hours later, I awoke to the phone ringing. Anu explained that they were at the ER at MCMC, and why.

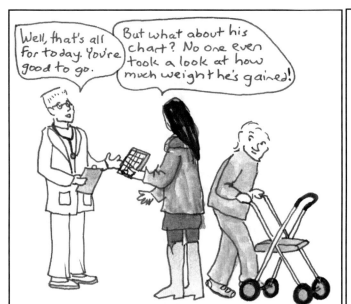

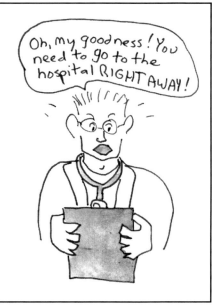

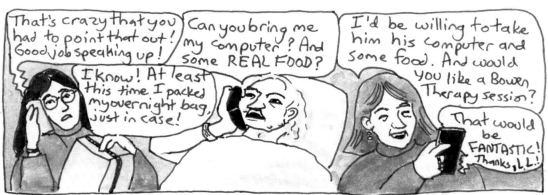

Thank goodness L.L. called me right after Anu and Aubrey called me! She was just checking to see how things were going. When she heard that I was planning to drive to the city to bring Aubrey's requests, she offered to do it for me. So I got to stay home with Earl and do some home-schooling. That also meant we were home when Aladdin brought more yummy meals from the cancer resource center volunteers. (I'd forgotten!)

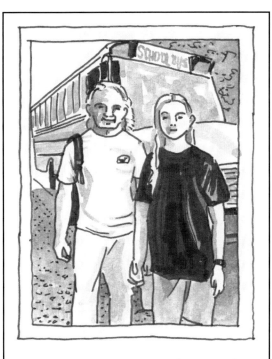

Support a Community Member in Need

~~~~

Update 1/30/17
Dear friends,

After a cheerful week at home and many visits with family and friends, Aubrey is back in the ER at MCMC with much fluid in the heart again, caused by a large tumor there and some in other places. In spite of this he is being the same mellow, fearless, cheerful guy you all know.

Besides paying old bills, your generous donations are helping with such needs as a $364 bottle of heart meds, a blood pressure cuff for taking readings at home, extra heating oil to keep the house at 70 degrees, gas money for his daughter to visit from two states away, and high quality dark chocolate for rewards because Aubrey is being such a good sport during all of these doctor visits. Thank you so much for all the love and support you've showered Aubrey with!

Eventually, Aubrey was checked into a room in the cardiology wing at MCMC, to spend the rest of the day under observation. When the cardiologist assessed him, and looked through the week's worth of various kinds of scans, she discussed how the growing tumor in the heart added to the pressure and fluid build-up. The tumor could not be removed without killing him, but having another drain put into his heart could buy him some time. It had helped once. Was he up for the risk of doing it again? He was all for it. There was some discussion of putting a permanent drain, called a "window," into the pericardium, so that the draining of fluid could happen as needed, without more invasive surgery. However, implanting the window itself was more of a high risk surgical procedure than making a temporary drain. The decision was made to just do the same procedure as the last time. They did it the next day, Tuesday, January 31st.

Wednesday, February 1st, a nurse or care manager from MCMC called me to say Aubrey was being discharged around noon, and that a home care nurse would be in contact with us soon. I asked if his urinal from the hospital could be sent home with him, and she said yes. Problem solved? No!

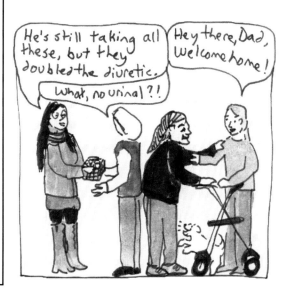

Things that go bump in the night:

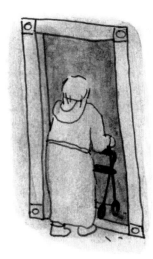

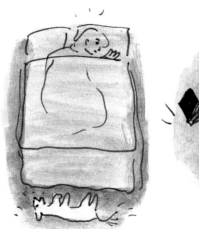

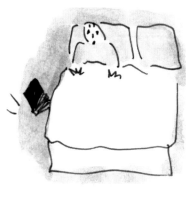

Rolling walkers going over thick door sills between rooms in old wooden houses every time some guy needs to walk between the bathroom and the living room.

Old diabetic dogs going blind and deaf who don't judge distances well anymore and sometimes fall off of beds or down the stairs.

Boys, awakened by dogs and dads, trying to distract themselves from thinking of death by reading books, who fall back asleep so the books may fall from their hands.

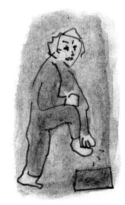

Moms trying to move quietly though creaky old houses to let old dogs out to pee, again, or check on the guy downstairs who seems to be awake a lot more now, maybe just doing yoga, or maybe passed out, having a heart attack, it might be good to go check. They creep to the edge of the stairs, stub their toes! Dang! Might as well have turned on all the lights!

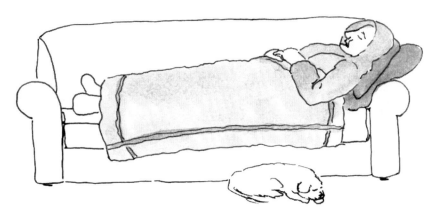

Increasingly, our household took to sleeping in and taking naps during the daytime to make up for such disturbances during the night.

Cancerous Fears

Cancer brings you face to face with mortality, particularly if you can see the tumors growing bigger and the body deteriorating, as Earl and I could when we looked at his dad. I worked to subdue a sense of alarm and disgust when viewing these tumors.

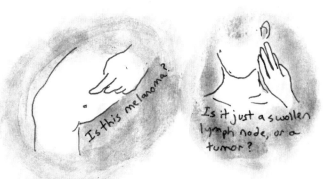

Perhaps the physical reflex to want to turn away and steer clear of that which is diseased and decrepit is a natural survival instinct, a way to avoid becoming contaminated by a thing oneself. Taking this reflex to a new level, some people believe they will "manifest" more of whatever they think about and focus on, positive or negative. If this were true, we were toast. We thought about cancer a lot. (We couldn't help but contemplate: what if some of the lumps, bumps, and dark spots on ourselves might also be tumors?)

Some people believe that people who are ill have "manifested" disease through their own "negative" thinking. This can lead to judging those who are enduring ordeals, blaming them for creating their own illnesses.

There were many ideas floating around on the Internet, particularly on Facebook, about alternative healing, natural healing, spiritual healing, mind-over-matter healing. It was mind boggling! Aubrey was already trying to apply many ideas to try to heal himself. I didn't want him (or any of us close to him) to be pressured by people's advice. So I explicitly told our community, through social media, that Aubrey was all set for ideas on how to treat, fight, manage, or fix the cancer, and that we were not shopping around for new ideas or advice. Fortunately, everyone respected this, and if they did have opinions, they politely kept them to themselves.

It takes courage, and willingness to look beyond the disease and the devastating changes it renders, to keep renewing connection, and being present with a very ill person. Illness challenges us to remember the person's true spirit and soul, to learn to see beyond the situation, while being immersed in the situation.

Such philosophical thinking is fine for an adult to contemplate, but it shouldn't be expected of a child. Earl was up late, two nights in a row, telling me he couldn't sleep because he felt anxious and depressed. He said overhearing medical talk freaked him out, and he asked for an overnight with Ella as soon as possible. I tried to comfort him, but agreed that his feelings counted as much as his dad's need for help. It was time to talk to Angela about other arrangements. Would Aubrey's insurance cover the nearby nursing home? She said it could take a while to get that sorted out, but she would start looking into it.

A New Hope?

Thursday, February 2nd, the day after he came home from the hospital, was Aubrey's first meeting with his oncologist. For this monumental event, both Anu and I went along. It was the meeting he had been looking forward to, and he was eager to discuss the possibility of doing immunotherapy.

When the oncologist lifted Aubrey's shirt and palpated his abdomen, I took a peek, then regretted it. There were lots of nubbly tumors on the skin, like dark button mushrooms growing from a log, and the skin was lumpy with internal tumors, like a sock full of blocks. The oncologist said that immunotherapy had a chance of helping. It could slow the growth of the tumors and even shrink them. Then he quickly listed a bunch of awful-sounding side effects, but said they could all be managed, and his tone of voice was brightly optimistic. I might have been dreaming, but I seem to remember hearing the words "a chance of recovery," and "months, even years." Suddenly angry, I subtly mouthed, "*WTF?*" to the nurse who was looking on. This feeling caught me by surprise.

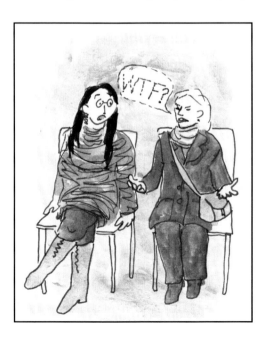

I wasn't against immunotherapy or chemotherapy, *per se*; two dear friends had been saved by the latter. When I tried to understand what the anger was based on, the only reason I could think of was that there seemed to be an incongruity between this doctor's perspective and everyone else's we had met on this journey so far. Professional people had been coaching me to make haste and prepare for The End: get a will in order ASAP; try to get Aubrey to sign the Do Not Resuscitate form; choose a funeral home or crematorium; take my kid to a counselor to talk about the approaching death of his dad. And now, there was a suggestion that Aubrey might sail into a bright new future of months–or even years! You'd think this would have made me feel happy for him, but it didn't, because I didn't believe it.

In my role as Aubrey's health care advocate, I asked: Wasn't there a possibility that this treatment might make him feel worse and weaken him faster than not doing it at all? I felt the response was patronizing in both tone of voice and vocabulary. Still, it was Aubrey's choice–and my role to uphold that choice. So, the first infusion was scheduled for a week later.

In the evenings, to disconnect from everything, I had been watching a sit-com. One comedic theme was that every scene with a medical professional was played by the same actor, and his screen name was always "Dr. Spaceman," pronounced "Spi-cheh-min." He was always outrageously under-qualified for whatever he was doing, yet pompously convincing, so everyone just went along with whatever he said to do, no matter how ridiculous it seemed. When I got home after that appointment and tried to recall what Aubrey's oncologist looked like, honestly, all I could picture was Dr. Spaceman. I'm not saying he was a bad doctor, in fact, Aubrey liked him and wanted what he offered. My reaction was my own issue to work on. It helped to talk with Angela, whose job it was to be a compassionate listener. She affirmed that my concerns were legitimate, but also coached me that it was Aubrey's choice and his decision to make.

Spin Control

Another moment of concern I felt at that appointment was about something I thought I heard the nurse say after the oncologist left the room. I heard the words "chemotherapy" and something about "secondhand exposure" and that there was some risk for people who were "immunocompromised."

Without the benefit of time for quiet reflection and composure, sensing the appointment was quickly drawing to a close, I blurted out, "Chemotherapy?! I thought immunotherapy was different! Less toxic! And *I am immunocompromised*! We need to get the doctor back in here to talk about this some more!"

Quickly, she recanted the word "chemotherapy." "Oh, I didn't mean 'chemo,' immunotherapy isn't the same as chemo; we just get used to calling it all 'chemo' since it all takes place up at the Infusion Center."

Oh. Silly me. I felt very foolish for overreacting.

Nurse Spin, as I shall call her, described that the treatment would wake up Aubrey's own immune system to pay attention to and attack the cancer cells, instead of ignoring them as it was now, so he is the one who would become immunocompromised, so people who were sick should stay away from him or wear masks. Because it engaged his own immune system, Aubrey saw this as working in a "natural" way, which is why he'd been open to trying it. I knew, from a bit of online research, that there were different kinds of immunotherapy, but I didn't understand the nuances enough to ask detailed questions with fancy vocabulary (and when I'd tried to ask I'd felt talked down to, as if I my questions were foolish and I misunderstood how the treatment worked). It was after 5:00 p.m., so the clinic was closing. Anu left, then Aubrey and I went to SBH for blood tests. By the time we got home it was late. After dinner I posted an update that was much more optimistic than I felt.

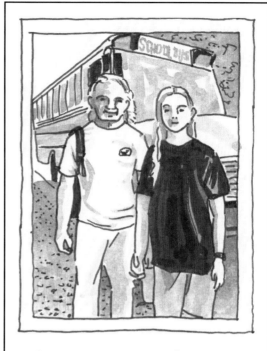

Support a Community Member in Need

~~~~

Update 2/2/17
Dear community,

As well as paying off outstanding medical bills your generous support is literally supporting us at a fundamental level of daily living while there is no other earned income by Aubrey and his ex-wife (who is hosting him).

Good news is that Aubrey got the green light from the oncologist to try immunotherapy this coming week! Aubrey is getting good rest now that he is back from a second stay in the hospital, and enjoying the home cooked food delivered by a group of wonderful volunteers who serve the cancer resource center.

Fluid and tumors around the heart still make it a very vulnerable situation. In spite of this, he is keeping a positive attitude and making progress writing his book.

Nurses Return

Friday, February 3rd, the visiting nurse returned, along with a new one. Between this visit and the one with the first nurse eight days earlier, Aubrey had been removed from that home care program, enrolled in Hospice's home care program, taken out of Hospice when someone somewhere deemed immunotherapy to be "curative," and then re-enrolled in the visiting nursing program! He was thus a "new" client, so they were here to orient us regarding the program, all over again! Everyone was somewhat confused about all this.

Aubrey seemed reluctant to engage with them, partly because they came when he was having a good streak of writing–not merely napping, eating, or shaving.

They described other services that could be provided through their program, such as Occupational Therapy and a visiting Social Worker. OT didn't seem necessary: Aubrey already had more conscientious use of his body than most people did, from all those years of yoga and hiking. He was already aware of, and doing his best, to work with the edema induced restrictions to his movement, by composing new yoga routines for himself in order to stay as limber and have as much balance and strength as possible. (In the distant past, he had actually taught yoga to others, in classes and private tutorials.) He didn't want someone in a suit telling him what to do. We didn't have a clue why a Social Worker would be necessary. We already had Angela. That left the nursing part. Aubrey was reticent to have any of it. He said he didn't need help with diet, blood pressure, medicines, shaving, eating, or bathing.

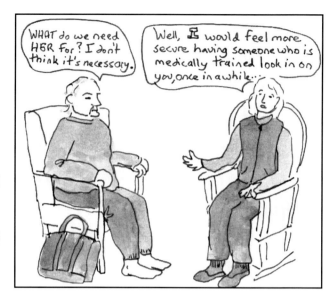

But I felt that having a nurse visit us once a week would be wise because she would become familiar with his symptoms, able to recognize if any changes were worthy of reporting, so that it was not all up to Aubrey and me to determine when to seek medical help or when to sit tight and be patient. He conceded my point, and agreed to let a nurse come once a week–at least for my sake. I showed them the open bucket and Mason jar rig, and requested a urinal, again. They explained they would not be visiting us again, but a urinal could be delivered by a different nurse who would be assigned to his case. She would visit within a week.

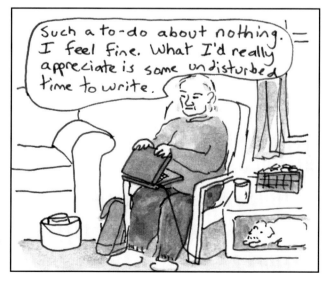

Too Much

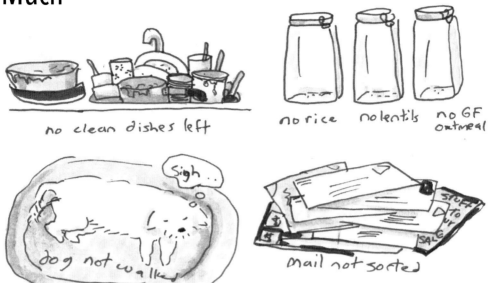

no clean dishes left

no rice   no lentils   no GF oatmeal

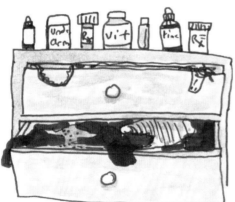

Sigh..

dog not walked

mail not sorted

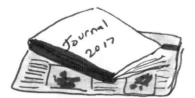

clothing not folded but at least in drawers

Journal not written in, newspaper not read

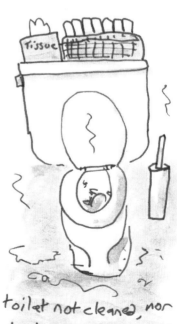

toilet not cleaned, nor bathroom floor, gross!

Coping Strategies

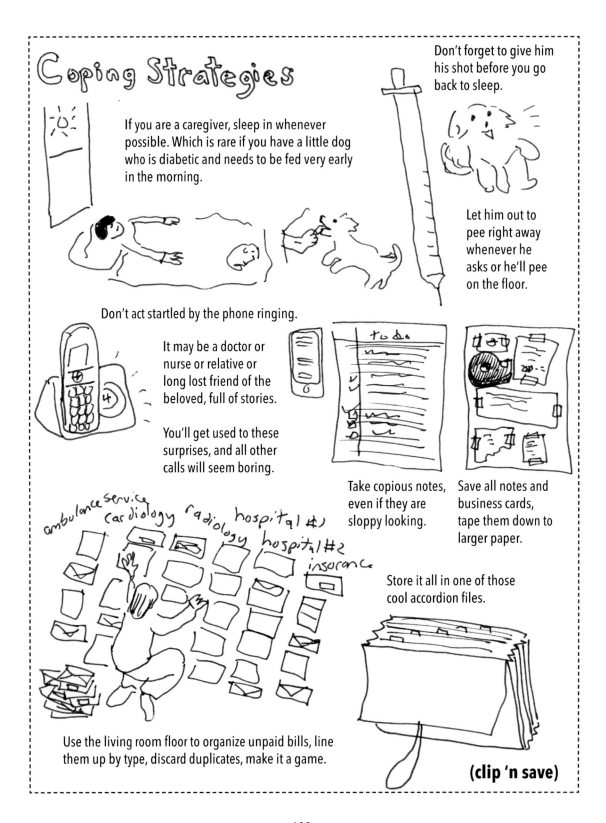

If you are a caregiver, sleep in whenever possible. Which is rare if you have a little dog who is diabetic and needs to be fed very early in the morning.

Don't forget to give him his shot before you go back to sleep.

Let him out to pee right away whenever he asks or he'll pee on the floor.

Don't act startled by the phone ringing.

It may be a doctor or nurse or relative or long lost friend of the beloved, full of stories.

You'll get used to these surprises, and all other calls will seem boring.

Take copious notes, even if they are sloppy looking.

Save all notes and business cards, tape them down to larger paper.

Store it all in one of those cool accordion files.

ambulance service cardiology radiology hospital #1 hospital #2 insurance

Use the living room floor to organize unpaid bills, line them up by type, discard duplicates, make it a game.

(clip 'n save)

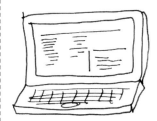

Let key people in on the story: your kid's teachers, principal, private lesson instructors, and coaches. Anyone who is cool will want to "have your back."

Wear your favorite clothes that are the most comfortable. Dress nicely enough that if you suddenly get a phone call and have to go to the ER or ICU or meet with doctors you will look as if you mean business.

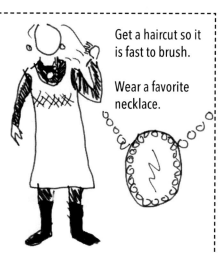

Get a haircut so it is fast to brush.

Wear a favorite necklace.

"Let us know if there is anything we can do for you."

"Of course he can turn it in late. Family comes first!"

"We are so sorry, please keep us in the loop so we can support him."

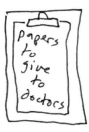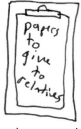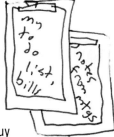

Use all the clipboards you own, buy more. (I used seven at one point.)

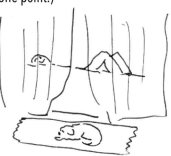

Have lots of baths. Add sea salt, or Epsom salts, or bubble bath, or a few drops of lavender oil.

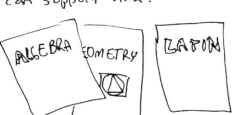

Don't sweat it if your child gets behind in every subject, but still encourage his or her accomplishments. It is impossible and absurd to be dogmatic in the face of the impending death of a parent.

(clip 'n save)

Go to bed early. Watch movies and read graphic novels. Eat dinner in bed, drink red wine.

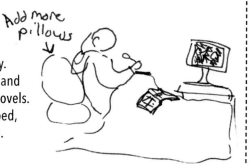

What about the rest of us?

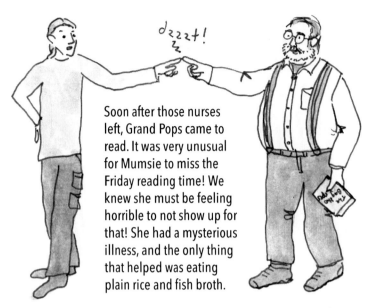

dzzzt!

Soon after those nurses left, Grand Pops came to read. It was very unusual for Mumsie to miss the Friday reading time! We knew she must be feeling horrible to not show up for that! She had a mysterious illness, and the only thing that helped was eating plain rice and fish broth.

Aubrey enjoyed the reading time, and after that he got his wish for quiet writing time. Glad to be done with all those pesky medical appointments and home visitations, he enjoyed the weekend working on his novel, interspersed with naps and hearty meals.

Steve stayed in The Big City for the weekend, as per my request. I was feeling too overwhelmed by the massive amounts of novel information, conversations, directions, schedules, and general turmoil to change tack and make merry with any house guest.

Anu spelled me for three hours on Saturday morning while I got out. She seemed to be holding up well, but she'd missed a lot of work and had to keep asking colleagues to cover her shifts. She was very concerned about Rhia, who was feeling a lot of angst about living so far away, unable to help her dad, wondering whether to quit her job and move back home, or not.

Certainly this must be a familiar saga for many people who are not living close to their ill loved one. No one could give Rhia any advice that was helpful. If she stayed put and held steady, she might miss the last days or weeks with her dad. But if she quit and moved, she might not find work, and he might die right away, or live for months. No one knew. The decision was hers, and there were no clear answers.

Ella was also under duress. I knew she was doing treatment for Lyme disease, but I hadn't realized how much she was struggling: as well as feeling achy and nauseated, she was also having a hard time reading and writing because of problems with short-term memory. That made doing college level work so difficult that she was considering taking a medical leave. Unfortunately, she wasn't getting much help or mothering from me, which I sorely regretted.

When a family member becomes critically ill, it's natural for that person's needs to become the focus of everyone around them. Those without life threatening conditions often take a back seat in terms of getting attention and support. This happens unconsciously, as everyone focuses on what seems most critical and forgets to check in with one another, and it happens consciously, when people deem their own problems to be less important because theirs are not life threatening. Out of politeness they may recede from drawing attention, or perhaps they believe there is not enough attention to go around, or that nothing can be done to help them, anyway, so they withdraw.

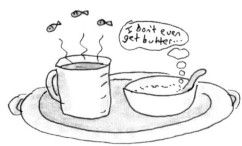

I don't even get butter...

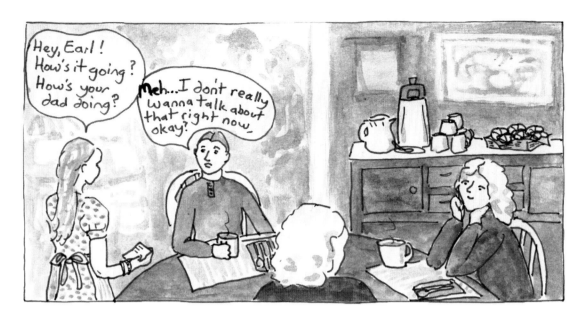

A friend of Aubrey's spelled me for a couple hours on Sunday morning so I could go out to breakfast with Ella and Earl. It had been too long since I'd had any quality time hanging out with both of my children. We decided not to talk about icky things, and instead focus on enjoying the meal, discussing anything light-hearted, comical, or interesting.

It was lovely being out at a restaurant, choosing food off a menu, and having someone else prepare it! The owners were friends who were aware of our situation at home. They kindly gifted us with the meal! (There are some advantages to living in a small town where everyone knows you.)

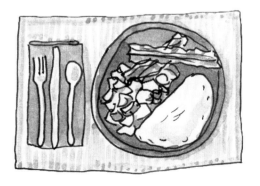

There are also some disadvantages. When out in public places, such as the restaurant, it was sometimes necessary to consciously protect our boundaries. When people know something big is going on with a person whom they care about, it is natural and even respectful for them to inquire. But it is also appropriate to decline comment or to delay these conversations until a more convenient or appropriate time. At MCMC, the Hospice liaison had coached us that it was okay to tell people we didn't want to talk about something; we could simply say, "Thanks for asking, but it's not a good time for me to talk about that."

Other than group emailing a few of my friends now and then, I was so deeply immersed in coping with the situation that I didn't want to talk about it yet. Explaining took too much energy. It was too big to wrap words around.

Although I was sharing some information via the fundraiser and Facebook posts, I was also holding back a lot, so most people had no idea how difficult things were on a very gritty physical level as well as emotionally. They also made assumptions, and had their own emotional reactions to work through. Some would get teary and sad, and I didn't feel up to holding the space for them. A restaurant most definitely was not the place to fill them in.

People can't help but make assumptions, based on the little they know, or in reference to their own experiences, which they deem similar to yours. For example, some people assumed that for Earl, having his dad "at home" full time meant he enjoyed a lot of sweet loving cozy father-son bonding time.

Earl could appreciate this assumption, conceptually. But what no one would understand unless living with us, was that it was odd for him to have so much domestic time with his dad. They were both used to meeting for walks and hikes, then retreating back into their privacy bubbles—not sitting around the table, chewing the fat for hours, day after day. It wasn't that they didn't talk, but a few well placed words were sufficient.

When they did come to the table for a "family" meal, there was mostly silence, except for the sounds of chewing, swallowing, and me making chirpy comments, trying to offer conversation starters. This new cohabitation situation did not suddenly turn father and son into loquacious conversationalists. When Aubrey was not eating he was napping or quietly focused on his writing. He often seemed mentally preoccupied, not eager to engage in dialogue, so I usually kept conversation to the functional basics.

As much as Earl loved his dad and knew we should help him out, he was feeling a lot of anxiety. All the medical details were creepy and frightening. He didn't want to be in the living room with the blood pressure cuff, the charts and pills, and the Mason jars of urine. He stopped practicing piano because it was in the living room.

Once in a while he worked on wood carving projects downstairs, but mostly he carved in his bedroom. (One might have assumed beavers lived in there.)

Home-schooling was slipping by the wayside. Our attention spans were minimal. Earl couldn't stomach doing lessons at the dining room table, from which he could see, hear, and smell the patient in the next room. Aubrey needed the doors between these rooms to be left open in order to use his walker to get to the bathroom, and whenever he napped he snored. Earl didn't like seeing him with his mouth gaping open. Smells of various kinds were starting to increase. Earl and I were both spending more and more time upstairs, in our own bedrooms.

Since Aubrey had come home from the hospital the second time, Earl had been begging to sleep over at Ella's or her dad's house whenever he could. They kindly obliged, but she was busy with college, and her dad was about to travel out of the country. Though I hesitated to call upon Ella, she was Earl's main confidante besides me and my main back-up for driving him to music lessons and classes at school on short notice.

The middle school principal and teachers were kind. Everyone knew Aubrey from when he had been a bus driver there years ago. They asked how he was feeling, and if there were anything they could do to help. I wasn't sure what to ask for, but it was nice knowing that people cared. They said it was fine if Earl missed school or didn't do his homework: family comes first.

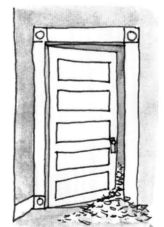

But Earl said school was one of the things he enjoyed the most. It got him out of the house, and gave him social time with people his age. It certainly wasn't the time for him to have friends over.

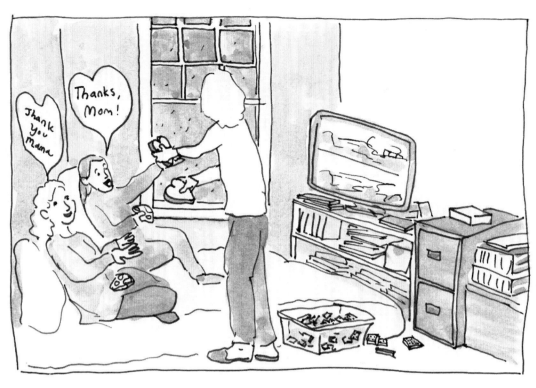

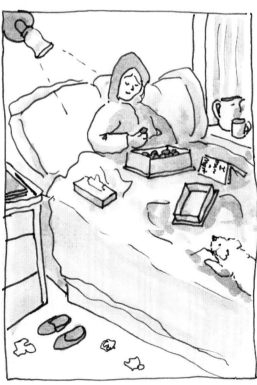

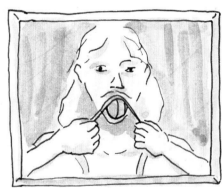

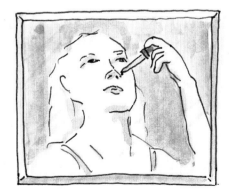

MORE Coping Strategies

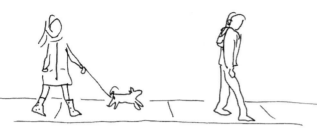

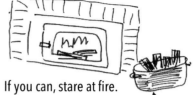

If you can, stare at fire.

Make your teen carry in the wood, exertion in small amounts can be grounding.

Take walks. Take walks together with family members who are also going through this ordeal, even if you are not walking side by side. Talking should be optional.

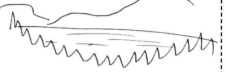

If you can, stare at water.

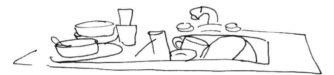

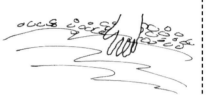

Accept messes. Inevitably there will be some long boring patches where there is no plot development in your family drama and you will become bored enough to be willing to clean up messes. Soon enough the phone will ring again, and then you'll have an excuse to drop everything and respond to the latest crisis.

Better still, go touch it.

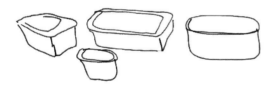

Let other people cook for you if they volunteer. Don't even think about how to repay them. You are in the trenches. Your time to be supportive to others in your position will come. (Thanks to my friends for the baked ziti and chocolate chip cookies and soup!)

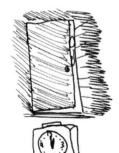

Let your kid come in and talk no matter how late or early it is.

Let him sleep in the next day.

Bring him breakfast in bed sometimes.

Other times, insist he come downstairs and eat with you.

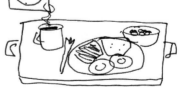

(clip 'n save)

A Week of Frustrations and Storms

Monday	Tuesday	Wednesday	Thursday	Friday
6 8:25 Art	7	8 Visiting (9:00) Nurse ?	9 8:25 French	10 8:25 French
~~12:30 E-Gid~~	~~12:45 Dr. Kay~~		11:00-2:00 1st Immunotherapy	
12:30 Food Delivery	(SNOW STORM!)	1:10-2:30 Social Studies	1:30-2:15 music lesson	
1:40-2:30 Soc. Studies	4:15 Vet		~~5:30-6:30 Fencing~~	1:10-2:30 S.S.
2:30 ECHO			(SNOW STORM!)	(SNOW STORM!) Steve by 8:30

After a quiet weekend of resting and writing, Aubrey had quite a line-up of appointments out in the world for the following week. It turned out to be a week of frustrations and storms.

Monday, February 6th, Anu drove forty minutes to town to take him to a 12:30 afternoon appointment at SBH. It was for an Echocardiogram, just like all those other times. The good thing was, some clever person had figured out he could do this locally, instead of driving to the city! The bad thing was, when they got to the clinic they were told that the appointment was for a different time and date! Everyone, including me, thought I must have written the wrong information on my calendar. This was very disconcerting. It had taken a lot of wind out of Aubrey's sails to get bundled up, push his walker through the snow to the car, then go into the hospital, then turn around and come back home. His breathing was labored and he was worn out. The good thing was, a new appointment was booked for 2:30 that afternoon. But Anu had to get back to her town to start her shift at the restaurant, and I had to get Earl from school, so I had to arrange for a friend to take Aubrey. After calling around to several people we found that The Farmer was willing and able, thank goodness! When he and Aubrey got to the hospital, they were told that the 12:30 p.m. appointment had been correct, after all! At least I was relieved that I wasn't so spacy as to have made that mistake.

The next day, Tuesday, February 7th, was supposed to be a check-up with Dr. Kay, but that appointment got canceled due to a snow storm. Oh well, just nature. The good thing was, we were relieved of the chore of going out into the storm, but the bad thing was, he'd been home from the hospital a week without a check-up, and was significantly gaining in water weight. Where was that visiting nurse we were told would contact us? It had been four days since our in-take meeting with the nurses in the living room, and no one had called to set up a visit with a new nurse. So, I called the number on the business card the other two nurses had left. An operator at a switchboard in a city far away said a new nurse was planning to come to the house the next day, Wednesday, February 8th. Say what? Why hadn't we been told? The way the system worked was that they waited until the day of the visit to contact clients. I complained that we would have no way to anticipate being home to meet a nurse without knowing at least a day in advance! After all, I had vet appointments, school appointments, and other events scheduled on my calendar, and Aubrey had been having so many appointments they'd be lucky to even find *him* at home! Oh well, that's just how the system worked.

In spite of worrying that it would look bad to complain, I couldn't just "let it go," so I started typing a letter of complaints, describing these frustrating situations.

What do we need HER for?

Wednesday morning, February 8th, the new nurse knocked on the front door.

"What do we need her for?!" Aubrey asked, again.

I quickly explained, all over again, what help she was here to provide.

Had he actually forgotten our prior discussion with the other two nurses, or was he just in a bad mood?

Was it just a mood, or was pain making him irritable?

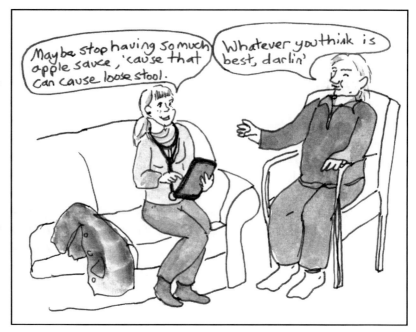

By the time her coat was off, he found it in himself to be welcoming and friendly. She confidently set about interviewing him, tapping information onto the screen of a hand held electronic device.

They seemed to be getting along nicely. I, however, looked at her and had a middle-aged, or "age-ist" moment, thinking, "She hardly seems old enough to have graduated from high school!"

Furthermore, she had not been given the message to bring a urinal! Apologizing, she promised to ask around and see if any of the other visiting nurses in the area might have one, and she would bring it to next week's visit.

Aubrey told her he felt no pain, and from his claims, sight unseen, one might conclude he should be able to live on his own. When he took a bathroom break, (without his walker, the show-off), I pulled Nurse Darlin' aside and filled her in on a few things.

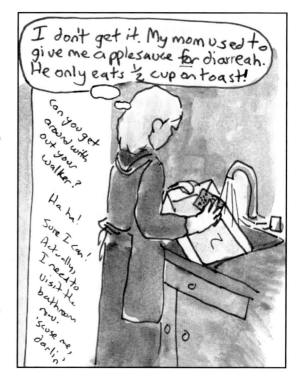

Shaving Accident

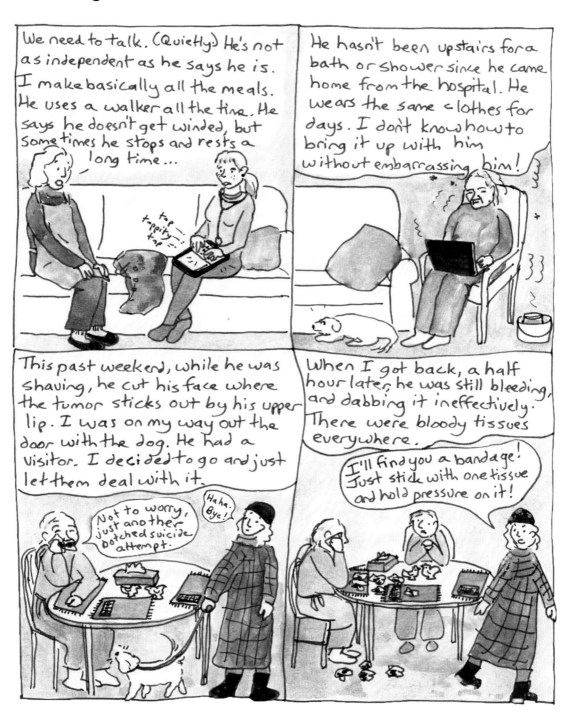

We need to talk. (Quietly.) He's not as independent as he says he is. I make basically all the meals. He uses a walker all the time. He says he doesn't get winded, but sometimes he stops and rests a long time...

tap tappity tap

He hasn't been upstairs for a bath or shower since he came home from the hospital. He wears the same clothes for days. I don't know how to bring it up with him without embarrassing him!

This past weekend, while he was shaving, he cut his face where the tumor sticks out by his upper lip. I was on my way out the door with the dog. He had a visitor. I decided to go and just let them deal with it.

Not to worry, just another botched suicide attempt.

Ha ha. Bye!

When I got back, a half hour later, he was still bleeding, and dabbing it ineffectively. There were bloody tissues everywhere.

I'll find you a bandage! Just stick with one tissue and hold pressure on it!

Being an Advocate

Aubrey was in the bathroom long enough so that I got to say everything that I wanted to say to the nurse in private. She nodded, said nice things to reassure me that she knew how nasty that must have been, and nimbly typed some more notes. When Aubrey got back to the living room, I was casually showing her his neat weekly charts.

She proved useful in several ways: consolidating pill taking from six times a day to four; giving us a big pill organizer which was easier and safer than the egg carton we'd been using; noting a significant weight gain, and calling it in to Dr. Kay, who authorized increasing the dosage of the diuretic.

As I heard her talking to Dr. Kay, I pointed out that the weight gain was even greater than she had calculated. What if I hadn't been listening in on her call to correct the math?

Why had it taken "the system" twenty-two days to send a visiting nurse to help us with critical issues such as accurate home-based pill taking?

I added these concerns, and the saga of the unobtainable urinal, to the letter of frustrations and complaints, then sent it off to what I imagined was "headquarters" at Small Brick Hospital.

That letter found its way to the desk of Mrs. Diplomacy, a patient advocate in the quality department, who mediated and resolved patient complaints. She replied with an invitation for me to call her. I did, not knowing what to expect.

She quickly set me at ease by thanking me for the carefully written information, apologizing on behalf of everyone, and agreeing that it all sounded very frustrating. She even thanked me for being a good patient advocate!

What does a Patient Advocate do?

There are professional Patient Advocates and Health Care Advocates, but a family member or friend might also help with these tasks:

- Accompany the patient to appointments.
- Take notes, or even record conversations, during appointments, to help the patient remember important information.
- Observe whether the patient is hearing and understanding all that the doctor and other officials are saying. If necessary, help "translate" complex information into words he or she can better comprehend.
- Be sure the patient's questions and concerns are addressed; if not, speak up.
- Ask any important questions the patient may have forgotten to ask or is too tired or compromised to think of asking.
- Find out what medicines the patient needs to take, how often, at what dosage, and what the common side effects are.
- Help the patient to self-assess whether there are side effects or other symptoms that warrant a call or return visit to a doctor.
- Help make appointments and remind the patient of them; arrange transportation.
- Help the patient prepare for appointments by gathering notes, charts, medications, and questions you or they have written.
- When problems or concerns arise, help the patient to figure out whom to talk to, or talk and write to others on his/her behalf.
- Help with paperwork at home.
- Help with banking, collecting mail, paying bills. (Find out what paperwork you both need to sign to give you permission.)
- Communicate with other family members and friends on behalf of the patient.

Who's Who at the Hospital

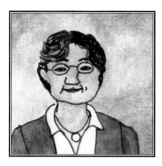

Clinical Social Worker

Does counseling, offers resources to patients and their families, focuses on inpatient needs but sometimes follows outpatients for a time as well.

In our story this is Angela's role. She first met us in the ER and helped us fill out important paperwork such as the Health Care Power of Attorney. She followed our case, so was handy to talk to when we were upset or confused while trying to address problems, but didn't know whom else to talk to or how to proceed in the system. She was trained to be emotionally supportive, and knew what other services were available, and connected us with other services and people as needed.

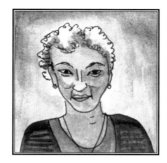

Patient Advocate

Works in the quality department, mediates and resolves patient complaints. Conflicts or complaints may start anywhere, and other people might try to resolve them, but if things get too sticky or involve other departments, this person can most quickly assemble the necessary people, and may serve as a facilitator during meetings.

In our story this is the role of Mrs. Diplomacy. When I wrote letters with problems and questions, she knew to whom to send them, arranged face to face meetings, and made sure we felt heard. She sent diplomatic follow-up letters regarding all issues.

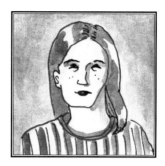

Social Worker

Specializes in connecting patients and their families with resources such as housing and Medicare. She makes home visits when necessary, takes referrals from the clinical social worker, from clinics that are associated with our hospital, and from the ER.

In our story this is Helpful Hazel's role. When I needed help filling out some health care forms and expediting their submission, she made a house call to explain some parts line by line, and while there made phone calls verifying some information. This made some confusing paperwork less overwhelming, and saved me another trip to the hospital, which meant not needing to line up a sitter at home.

Infusion Confusion

Thursday, February 9th, was Aubrey's first much anticipated immunotherapy infusion, at the Infusion Center at Small Brick Hospital. There was yet another snow storm, and Anu's car broke down, so I drove him there.

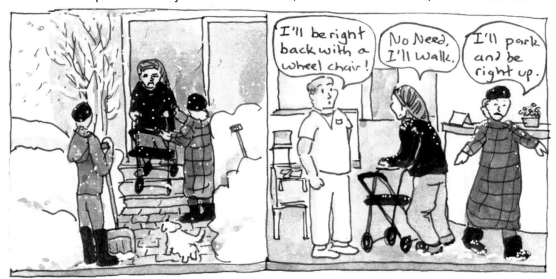

Since his blood work showed anemia, they added an IV of iron to the agenda, which meant he would be tethered there for almost three hours. He seemed fine being left to drift, so I left him in the hands of Nurse Spin. I also needed to get home to make lunch, shovel snow, walk the dog, and drive Earl to a music lesson, so I didn't linger to ask any questions.

When Aubrey was finished they called me and I drove right over. The nurse handed me a packet of papers describing side effects in detail, what to report, and a handout about home care. It explained that the patient's bodily fluids were considered hazardous for the first 48 hours after the infusion, especially for people who were immunocompromised.

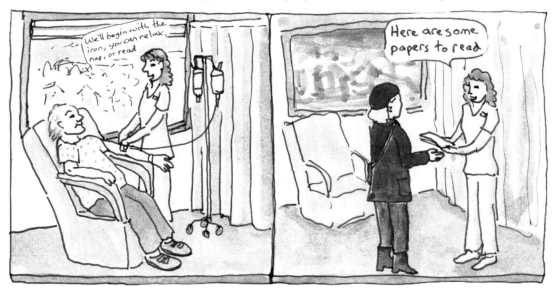

Ha! So I *hadn't* imagined hearing this at the oncology appointment! And I *wasn't* foolish for asking to discuss it further! (Please excuse me for a moment.)

I was astonished that this critical safety information was not provided on paper, and discussed up front, at any time *before* the infusion took place!

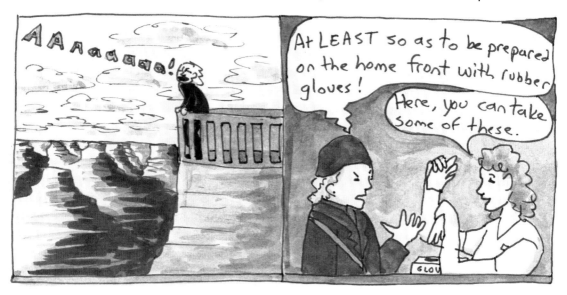

When I got home I texted Angela. She made an appointment for me to rant–I mean, for us to talk–at the hospital the next morning. As I was planning to explain to her, I was at risk. When an immune response got triggered, my body tended to over-react, and any inflammatory response took a longer time than normal to settle down.

My nervous system might also get ramped up. To avoid triggering an episode, I minimized exposure to sick people, crowds, and mostly worked from home. Usually I didn't talk about this, but now that I was at risk, it seemed important to confide in her. But that meeting never happened, because Angela didn't make it to work Friday morning!

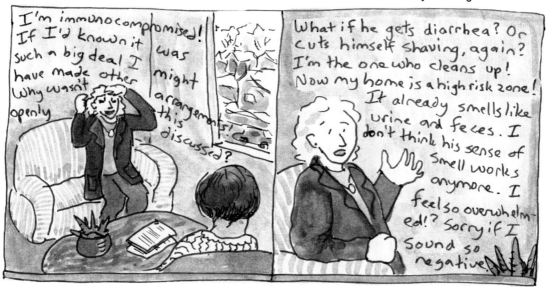

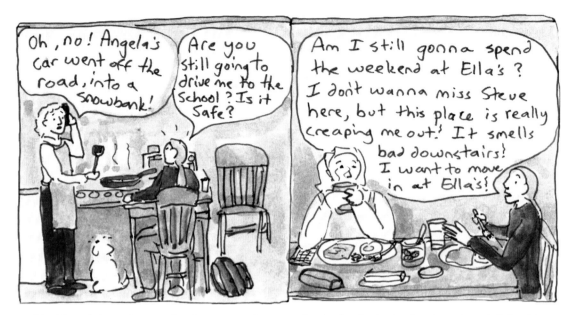

Earl had heard about the new development in the plot. I couldn't NOT tell him; his health was at risk too. He was eager to get off the main stage and take refuge at his sister's apartment.

After he finished school and we shoveled the driveway (again), Ella picked him up for the weekend. She kindly offered to let him sleep over any time it worked for their mutual schedules.

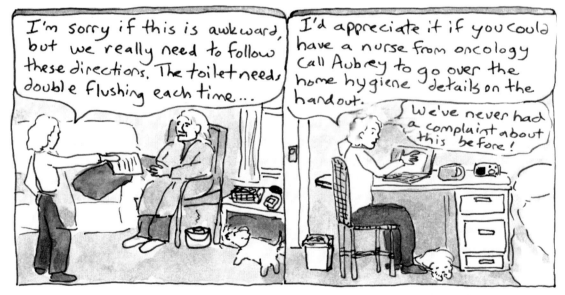

Aubrey said he would read all the handouts, but later in the day the toilet still needed flushing and there were spills on the living room floor. I didn't want to sound like the nagging ex-wife, so I called the clinic and asked for professional backup.

They told me it was standard procedure to give patients home care handouts after their first infusions. I questioned this, and wrote another complaint letter to Mrs. Diplomacy, and texted Angela, who passed along my concerns to others on duty at the hospital.

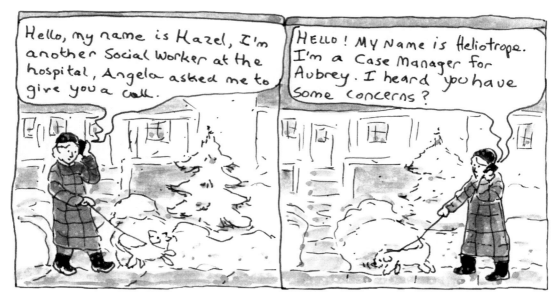

Hazel said that a social worker would be sent to visit us at home, some time in the following week. She reassured me that Aubrey would most likely qualify for long term care at a nursing home. We just needed to do more paperwork!

"Case Manager?" What a Good Idea! How had we not heard of her until a month into this drama? It was About Time Someone Was Managing Our Case!!! Anyway... I described some of the problems, such as not having a urinal yet, and why it was so important.

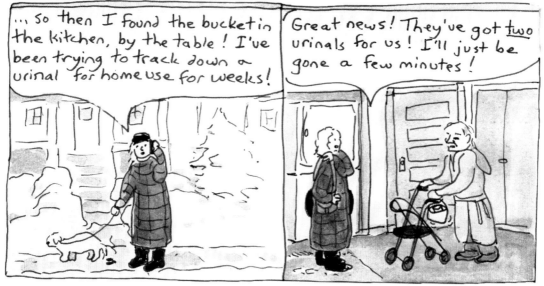

Owing to some expanding tumors "down there," aiming was becoming difficult. Not to worry, assistance was available: Heliotrope must have had some pretty high-up connections, because within minutes she tracked down not only one, but TWO urinals!

She said if I could come swing by Dr. Kay's clinic the marvelous urinals would be waiting for me in a bag at the front desk! Faaan-Tastic! Off I drove to pick them up.

While I was out, a nurse called Aubrey. She said it was HIS job to clean up all the messes he made, especially any on the floor. She was obviously oblivious of the fact that he could barely squat or bend over! I felt so bad!

We agreed he'd do his best to be sanitary, and I'd help clean. I washed my hands several times an hour, all day. That evening, Steve arrived for a romantic weekend with his zombie girl friend.

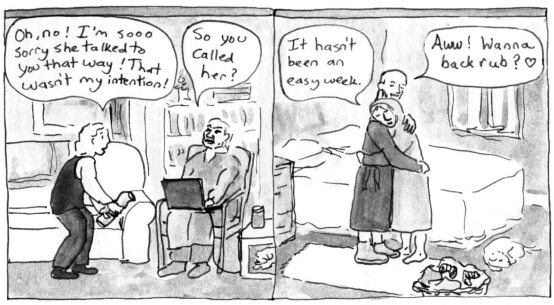

Snow fell through Saturday. Steve helped shovel. Aubrey's car got hidden under a big mound of snow. Earl and Ella called to check in. They were excited to be house bound, cozy in pajamas, watching movies.

Sunday Steve left early, to avoid getting stuck in the wrong state. By evening there was too much snow to safely drive, so Earl stayed at Ella's a third night. That was just as well. I was feeling under the weather.

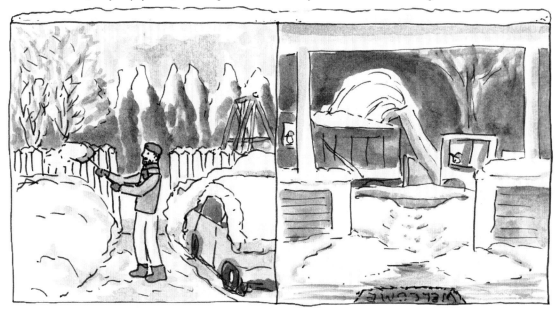

Monday, February 13th, was an official Snow Day off from school, a twelve hour blizzard. I was glad Earl was still at Ella's because my fatigue gave way to a low fever. I also felt spacy, tipsy, and dizzy.

Aubrey and I were in a pickle. Being sick, I wasn't supposed to be near him, but there wasn't any back-up for my role. It didn't feel right to ask any of our friends to put themselves at risk. The storm raged on.

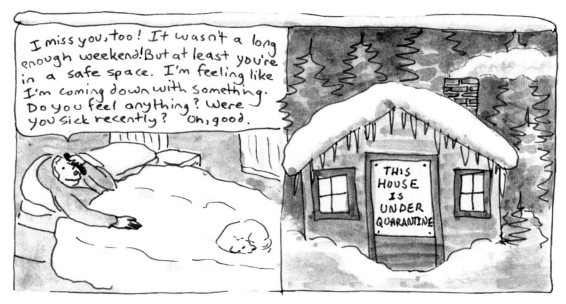

Things got worse overnight. I couldn't sleep. A rash like a sunburn spread from my neck to my chest and down my spine. My nervous system was on red alert. Whenever I stood up, I felt dizzy. It was like riding a tilt-a-whirl while on caffeine! It felt like my immune system was being kicked into overdrive.

Steve wasn't sick, nor had he been before his visit. No one else had visited us in a week. My children weren't coming down with a cold or flu or rash. When business hours started in the morning on Tuesday, I called and made an appointment to see my doctor that afternoon.

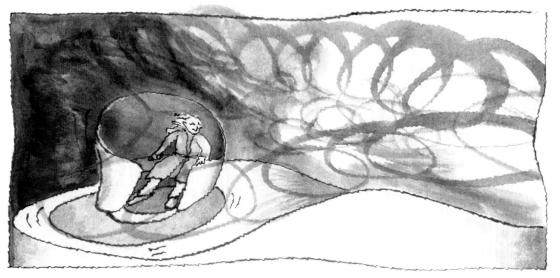

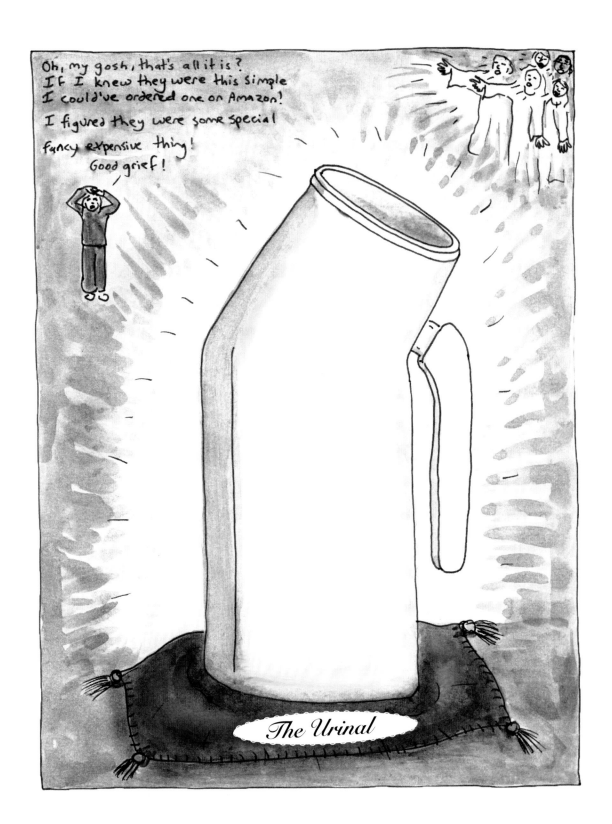

The Urinal

Some Parables of Unclear Thinking

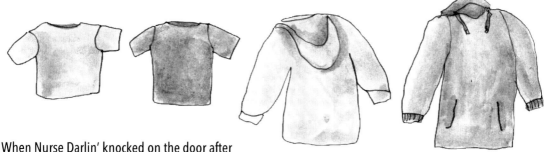

When Nurse Darlin' knocked on the door after breakfast that morning, I was so relieved to see her! Aubrey was still upstairs finishing his shower, so I had a chance to pull her aside and fill her in on a few things before he returned to the living room.

"Until this shower, he was wearing the same clothing since you were here last time! I asked what clothing he'd like to change into so I could carry it upstairs for him: I showed him two choices of short sleeved T-shirts, and two hooded sweatshirts, and asked which combination he wanted. He chose both hooded sweatshirts! I explained that two hoods might feel too bulky, and suggested he pick just one, plus a T-shirt to go under it. He seemed flummoxed by all this decision making, and asked me to make the choice for him.

"He's been spacing out on pill taking. Now I have to go in and give them to him at the right time, I can't just set them out and expect him to remember, not even for a half an hour.

"Then there's the issue of his mail. He wanted to give me his P.O. box key, and asked me to get his mail. I explained, for the third time, that we already set up to have his mail forwarded here. That's been set up for a month now, but to him it was news!

"He'll probably tell you he's feeling fine, but those are some examples of impaired memory and cognitive function since you were last here."

Sure enough, when Aubrey returned to the living room, he told her he was feeling okay–just a little diarrhea, more weary, and less appetite than usual. As she went down the list of immunotherapy side effects with him, I listened from the kitchen. The list contained many symptoms I was experiencing.

After she left I followed the directions on the immunotherapy home care handout: double bagging his dirty laundry in garbage bags, while wearing rubber gloves, then washing it separately. Then I scrubbed the bathroom floor, where his clothing had lain, and the upstairs sink, toilet, and tub.

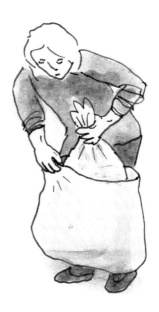

In Over Our Heads

Before getting to the doctor, I had to shovel a path from the back door out to the garage. There were well over four feet of snow, with mounds and drifts almost over my head! Thankfully, my kind old neighbor had a snow blower, and he'd already cleared the space between my garage and the road.

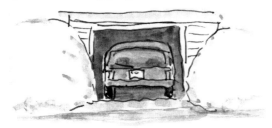

Also, there was a mound of new paperwork to complete on Aubrey's behalf: fourteen pages, to be exact; an application for nursing home care which Helpful Hazel had emailed to me the day before. One part needed to be finished by the bank, which I visited on the way to the clinic.

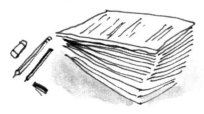

My doctor listened to me complain about my symptoms, which now included dizziness, a fiery feeling in the head, spine, and joints, some itchy sore spots on the skin, a runny nose, and no appetite. She was very sympathetic, but there was nothing to be done but wait it out. Then I explained about Earl not wanting to live at home anymore, asking to move in with his sister or her dad (but he was about to travel), how it was becoming harder to meet all of Aubrey's needs at home, the immunotherapy contamination risks going forward, and so on. She listened, then asked if I wanted to meet with Helpful Hazel, in person, right then and there! Excellent idea, I agreed!

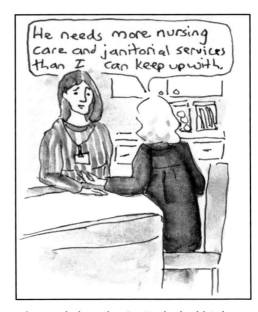

Hazel reminded me that Dr. Kay had told Aubrey that immunotherapy would only be palliative, not curative. I described to her how enthusiastically the oncologist had acted, as if he had not gotten that message himself. Hazel said she could help by getting Dr. Kay and the oncologist together in the same room, and that a "care team" was being assembled. The paperwork for the nursing home and insurance should soon be processed, so soon there should be more suitable accommodations for Aubrey.

Back home I started typing up a memo of everything I had discussed with Hazel, in order to provide everyone involved with an eye-witness view of Aubrey's decline in the past month, the different perspectives we were dealing with, anecdotes to back up my concerns about his problems and needs going forward (such as the examples of memory and cognitive impairment), and examples of how he needed more help than I could provide at home.

Aladdin came by with a new food delivery, and a friend of Aubrey's brought us some decadent homemade desserts. Even though I didn't feel like eating, these kind gestures and fine food made life briefly feel festive; it was Valentine's Day, after all!

Even though Aubrey and I weren't hungry, it was time to get dinner ready; Earl was coming home for the night. Ella had a date, was busy with her school work, and needed a break from playing sister-mom. They both had classes early the next morning.

Conceptually, I was operating from the belief that I was not sick with a communicable bug, but was on a wild ride of an immune system gone haywire, so I didn't try to avoid being in the room with Earl. Aubrey's conception was that I either had a bad bug, in which case I should stay away from him, or, that I'd been contaminated by him, in which case I should also stay away from him. He felt bad either way.

Like it or not, we needed to talk about the next phase: the nursing home. Since starting immunotherapy, Aubrey had turned a corner: from not believing he needed more care, to realizing that we were both in a compromised and precarious situation. I told him about my talks with Helpful Hazel, and that all the applications were finally finished. He agreed that the nursing home seemed sensible.

That evening, there was no emotional flurry of words between us that pushed me over the edge. There was more of a silent eruption within my mind, a private moment of losing all patience, as I proof-read the memo I was writing, one more time, and saw the absurdity of the situation we were in: I was in way over my head. We both were. My health was still tanking, and there was no telling how long until that would become resolved. Meanwhile, Aubrey's risk of developing internal bleeding, skin sores, ulcers, chronic diarrhea, and other common side effects, was only going to increase the longer he continued to receive more immunotherapy treatments.

Our son was vulnerable: anxious about sleeping at home in his own bed, and dependent upon at least one parent to remain available to take care of him. That thought might have been the one that tipped the balance. Up in my bedroom, I texted Angela.

"I can't take much more of this! My health is tanking, my child is at risk, if a room at the nursing home is not available for Aubrey this week, I'm just going to drive him over to the ER and leave him there for The System to deal with! It shouldn't be my responsibility to have to hold all this together!"

She responded. "You've done enough! You're done. Call 911 for an ambulance and send him to the ER. We'll take it from there."

Waves of relief.

Then the imagined images: bright flashing lights of an ambulance racing toward our house, pulling up right under Earl's bedroom window; neighbors looking out their windows, wondering what was going on; Earl's last memory of his dad at our home always and forever being of a stretcher rolling out the front door, right past the Christmas tree, which I still hadn't taken down.

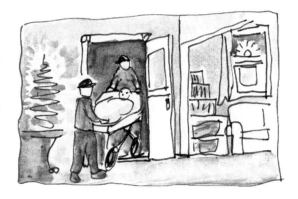

Nope. That was not how this scene should end! Besides, the front walk was only shoveled wide enough to let the mailman walk through. It wasn't prepared for a medical evacuation.

Texting Angela back, I said I could handle one more night, that it would be less traumatic and dramatic for all of us if I brought him over in the morning. She called me and we talked for a few minutes until I felt calm enough to go tell Earl and his dad the plan.

Last Fire

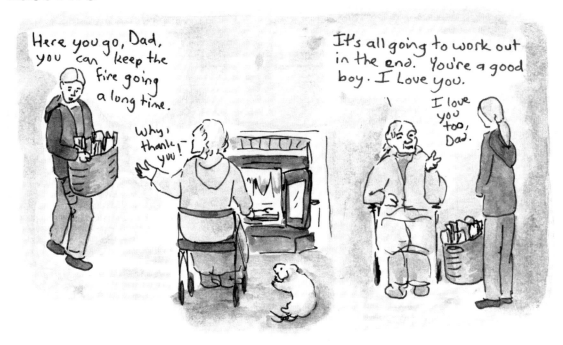

Sometimes it becomes too hard to keep a patient home, even if you love him and try as hard as you can. Even when you recognize you're in over your head, the heart pulls. You're worried about giving up on him, even if you know that it's in everyone's best interests to let go. This ambivalence is part of the journey.

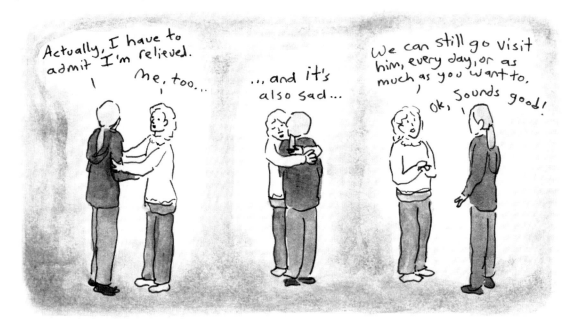

Facebook post Wednesday, February 15 at 9:58pm:

Update on the home front: made it through a full month with Aubrey here, Jan 14 - Feb 14, minus 8 days he was in the hospital, which were still totally "on" days for me driving to visit, staying overnight in the hospital hotel, doing mounds of paperwork and cleaning. On spiritual adrenalin I pulled off being full time nurse, janitor, cook, legal clerk, medical and financial power of attorney; got unpaid bills paid and two years of paperwork organized in folders, will filled out and witnessed, and turned in applications for state insurance, disability, and nursing home care.

Front row seat at this circus gave me privileged view of the "big picture" others were not seeing. Using my writing and advocacy skills sending memos, fielding a multitude of phone calls, I tried to connect dots between two hospitals, three clinics, disjointed contact from Hospice and Home Care, visiting nurses, visiting relatives, and visiting friends. Many kind and intelligent people, working in less than optimal systems of paperwork, protocols, and by-the-book procedures, caused mishaps in scheduling what, where, when, which led to frustrating delays in getting simple needs met, snow added further fettering, lack of back up began to pile up mentally and physically.

Possible second hand exposure to immunotherapy chemicals or possibly just the stress took my own health into a downward spiral of immune system on red alert, dizzy, head spinning, flushed feeling, itchy skin, no appetite, hypersensitive to sounds, smells, tired-wired insomnia; all just too much, and our son moved out for five days because it was all too much, so today I stopped trying to make it all work out, served Aubrey his last breakfast, made him a paper bag lunch, drove him to the ER, and left him in the hands of the social workers to find a room and figure out how to expedite nursing home placement because I've done what I can and perhaps more than I should have.

So the tide turns toward resting, sanitizing surfaces, staring into space, abandoning all identities and service roles other than Mom and home school guide, and not trying to keep anyone up to date on anything for a while.

Final positive closing statement: it was, overall, beautiful, because love prevailed. Aubrey's attitude of gratitude prevailed. Another unique precious chapter got lived together, and it's so clear that all the physical world is just the drama on the stage by which to learn that only love is real.

4.

Serenity Shores

Cleaning and Clearing

Visions of abandonment crowded my mind as I set about scrubbing floors: unwanted cats and dogs left on doorsteps in the dark of night, memories of telling Aubrey to move out while we were still married, and a warning from someone we knew who did elder care.

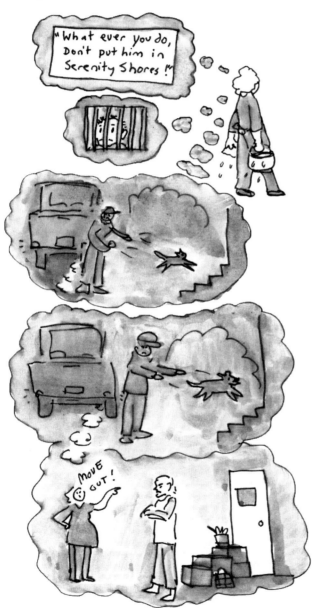

But each time these thoughts circled my mind, I reviewed the basis of the decision. It helped to know I wasn't alone in going through this process; remorse or even guilt is common for families to face when a loved one develops needs beyond their capacity to handle and an institutional home becomes necessary.

Perhaps if he had opted out of treatment, accepted Hospice and palliative care, had a real hospital bed with a raised back, a Hospice nurse or volunteer visiting daily, and easy access to a full bathroom on the first floor, we could have pulled it off. Or, looking back with hindsight, perhaps the way things fell apart, catalyzing the move, had a silver lining: making us move him into professional care before things became even more difficult.

On the short drive to the hospital that morning Aubrey had seemed mellow and accepting. In fact, he may have been secretly relieved to not be so much of a burden on his family. He even told Earl that visits should be considered optional, only if and when Earl felt like it.

This advice stemmed from his belief that he would miraculously rally, and from his experience with his own dad, who had gone into the hospital when Aubrey was fifteen. His mother and brother faithfully made frequent visits, but Aubrey didn't want to go. He didn't like seeing his dad so ill, nor to be in that institutional setting. His dad let him off the hook, saying, "It's fine if you don't want to come here, I understand, I don't blame you!" Aubrey repeated this story to Earl.

Earl said *of course* he would visit, and soon. He had more of a grasp of the reality of approaching death than his dad. We discussed this from time to time, and we accepted that if this was Aubrey's way of coping, we could respect that.

As soon as I felt up to it, I cleaned the downstairs floors, and any surfaces Aubrey had touched, three times over with soap and bleach, re-purposing the white plastic pee bucket as a wash bucket. Then the house felt safe for visitors. But every time I looked into the living room, the impression of it as a sick ward was still intact. Although the couch and chair were in good shape and clean enough, they would forever remind us of when that was "Dad's Bed" and "Dad's Chair." It was also the couch I'd purchased when Aubrey and I had moved in together years ago.

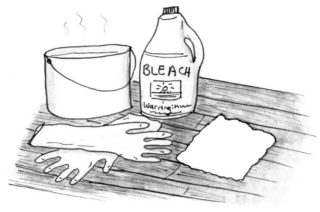

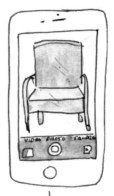

So many associations! The room needed clearing, as well as cleaning. I advertised both pieces of furniture, priced for quick sale. Earl and I lit candles and spritzed the room with nice smelling essential oil sprays to clear the air. Floating around on the Internet were ideas on "clearing negative energy" from a space, but that way of looking at it seemed to make the situation more dramatic than it needed to be.

While it seemed important to acknowledge the associations, and to recognize that Aubrey moving out was the end of an era, it seemed better to give the room a "blessing" to start out fresh, rather than a "purging" of "negative" energy. On our own, each in our own way, Earl and I said prayers and set intentions for the room to seem neutral again, a space to host warm cozy gatherings for family and friends.

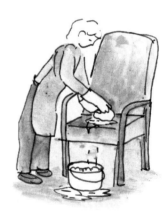

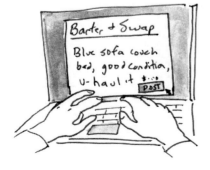

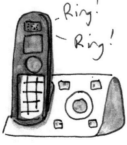

Within a short while, both the couch and the chair found new homes, and the half empty living room had a period of "chilling out" when we didn't go in there at all.

Pit bull and others to the rescue!

Fortunately Anu's car was fixed in time for her to go to Aubrey's one week follow-up appointment with Dr. Spaceman, Thursday, February 16th. I was still in no condition to be out and about, nor in a mood to hold polite conversation, at least within that context. I felt profoundly exhausted, and flatline emotionally, as well as a dizzy caffeinated whirl. When she stopped back at my house to pick up some of Aubrey's books and clothes along with a sandwich he'd requested, she reported that the oncologist hadn't even done a physical exam, but had claimed, cheerfully, that the tumors might already be shrinking from the first treatment! Well, I had to give it to the man, that was some powerful positive thinking! We rolled our eyes but conceded that it didn't hurt for Aubrey to have some hope. He planned to have infusions every three weeks. I worried about the increasing risk of side effects with each treatment; he seemed to have gotten his appetite back, and enjoyment of food was part of what small quality of life he had left.

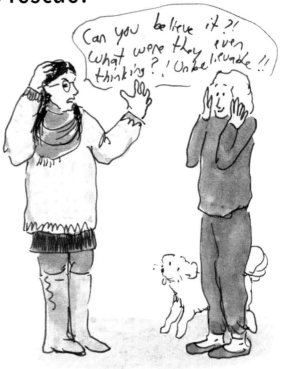

The next day, Anu continued to be heroic. Apparently Aubrey did *not* qualify for the local nursing home, based on an interview he had with the state's insurance program. (At over a hundred dollars per day to live in the cheapest local nursing home, we really couldn't afford it unless insurance could help cover it.) Apparently, he was so independent that the only place he qualified for was a group home for independent elders, off in another city, far away from all of his family and friends, and much too far away for daily sandwich deliveries! Of course we understood that if anyone really knew how things were, they'd understand that this made no sense! Anu figured out that when Aubrey was interviewed he must have once again overestimated his abilities. She spoke up and pulled what she called her "pit bull" act, adamantly demanding that "the powers that be" reconsider. She made phone calls and talked to people at the hospital about his infirmities, drawing anecdotes from the copious notes I had emailed to her.

By the time she left the hospital to go to work the dinner shift, she'd managed to make sure that everyone could see that Aubrey was indeed eligible for nursing care at Serenity Shores!

Meanwhile, a friend of mine came by the house and gave my head and spine a cranial sacral treatment, which took the edge off the dizzy whirling feelings. Grand Pops read to Earl, and Mumsie brought us a full Thanksgiving dinner, with roast turkey and all the classic side dishes, which we ate on trays in bed.

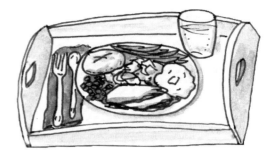

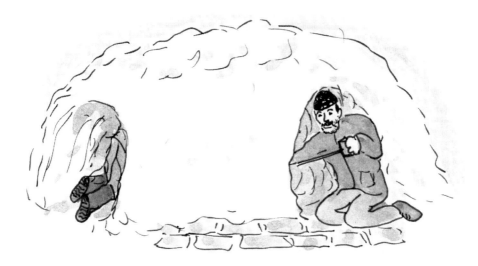

Late that night, Steve arrived for a long weekend. He had Monday off, due to it being President's Day. All day Saturday he cooked, cleaned, shoveled snow with Earl, stuck steel wool into holes in the basement ceiling so mice couldn't come up to the kitchen, and then we all watched movies in bed and ate popcorn for dinner!

Sunday, February 19th, was the first day I felt somewhat closer to normal. After brunch at our favorite restaurant, Steve accompanied Earl and me to our first visit with Aubrey, who had at last gotten a room at Serenity Shores. We were very curious to see inside the place, having never visited anyone there before. It was a place one would drive past on the way to somewhere else, until one knew someone who had moved in.

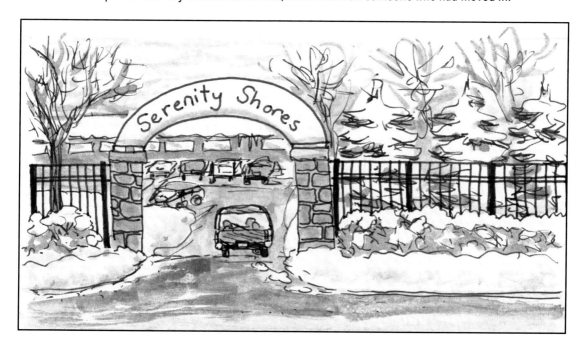

Serenity Shores

Serenity Shores was an old mansion on a lake, with two modern wings spread out to the east and west. Aubrey was in the east wing, which was for residents with more mobility and less need of intensive nursing care. There was always a night nurse on duty, and there were daily check-ins with The Matron. The Cook planned all the meals, helpers cleaned bathrooms and did laundry, and nurses assisted with taking pills on time (or at least within an hour of when they were supposed to be taken.)

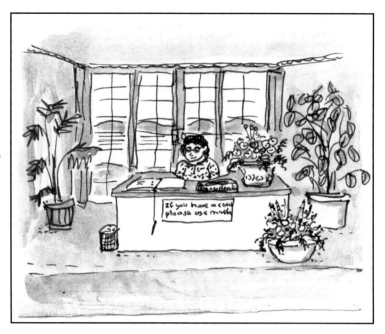

When we visited, we would sign in at the front desk in the lobby and proceed unaccompanied to his room. Sometimes the front desk was decked out in massive bouquets of fresh flowers. Sometimes the flowers weren't quite as fresh, and sometimes there were no flowers. We suspected these arrangements might be hand-me-downs from recently vacated rooms or even funerals. (Recycling is good, in any case.)

Aubrey was so happy to see us! We brought a home cooked lunch with dark leafy greens, at his request.

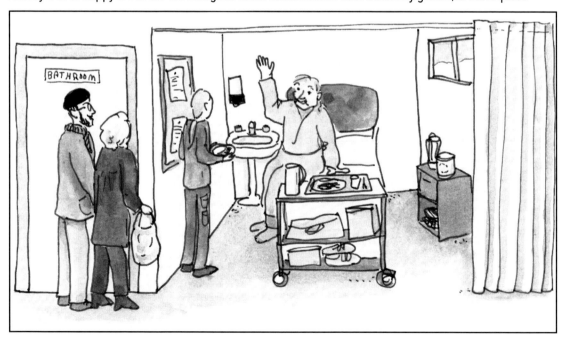

Aubrey shared a room and bathroom with another gentleman. Even though he probably preferred a solo room, he was lucky to have gotten in the door so soon, and this situation had some charm because long ago his roommate's son had been on Aubrey's bus route, so the man recalled him with fondness. For a normally reclusive person, Aubrey sure was turning out to have a lot of connections! He didn't seem to mind having company, and besides, the man was often out of the room, down the hallway, sitting in a common space. Aubrey was often absorbed in his writing; he said he was making progress almost daily. He appreciated having a bathroom right around the corner from his bed; he could access it quickly even without his walker.

If he felt like doing so, he was free to walk down the hallway to the dining room and look through the big glass windows out to the fabulous view of the lake. A bald eagle could often be seen flying there. It really was a lovely setting, a better view than most folks have at home.

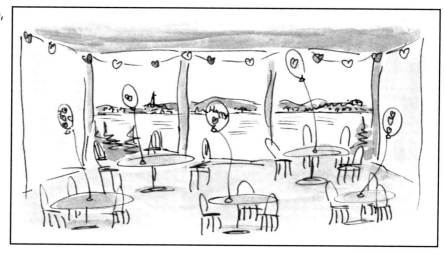

Rhia and Anu were mildly appalled by the lack of sterility in the institution, and I admitted I needed to hold my breath sometimes. (Strong cleaning compounds tend to point a finger at what they are made to conceal, and the old wall-to-wall carpet didn't help.) But I thought the dust and glitter under his bed from a former occupant was no more grungy than any of Aubrey's solo apartments had been over the years, and, putting it frankly to Anu and Rhia, I suggested that the place actually reminded me of some of his colorful writing. I even thought Aubrey himself might be aware of this, and see the place as "having character."

Every time we visited, the door to the shared bedroom was wide open. A parade of interesting people walked to and fro: nurses and doctors making rounds, people pushing carts loaded with trays of warm food or bins of laundry, custodians, visitors, and the residents themselves.

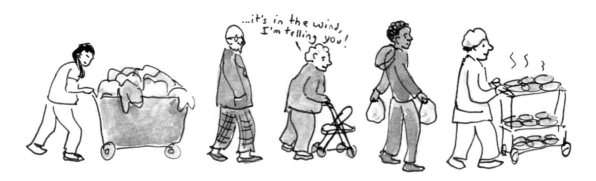

Many residents had some degree of dementia, and Aubrey had a deep well of patience and even a friendly interest in each one, as demonstrated by the way he never failed to greet all wanderers with enthusiasm and to participate sincerely in casual conversations with them—even if it were the same conversation every time. Reports of Baby Jesus having appeared at breakfast (and leaving foot prints!), cryptic sentence fragments uttered with deeply imploring eyes, were all met with active displays of interest on his part, as if there might be some deep prophesy or fortune-cookie-esque wisdom to be decoded from their words. He overlooked the soil and senility, and saw right through to a person's soul. Thus, he quickly became popular with the nurses and the residents.

It was a relief to me to find that the new living situation was actually working out all right for Aubrey. My function changed to bringing food that he liked (to augment what was served), and to running errands for such items as razor blades, new ink cartridges for his favorite blue fountain pen, and buying a mini-fridge. I kept visits brief, but he knew he could call me any time, and he frequently did. Talking over the phone brought back a nice sense of familiarity, for most days his voice was as sonorous and strong as it had always been. Earl didn't visit as much as I did, but whenever he asked I took him. (And sometimes I finagled excuses to bring him, such as needing him to carry the heavy box with the new mini-fridge).

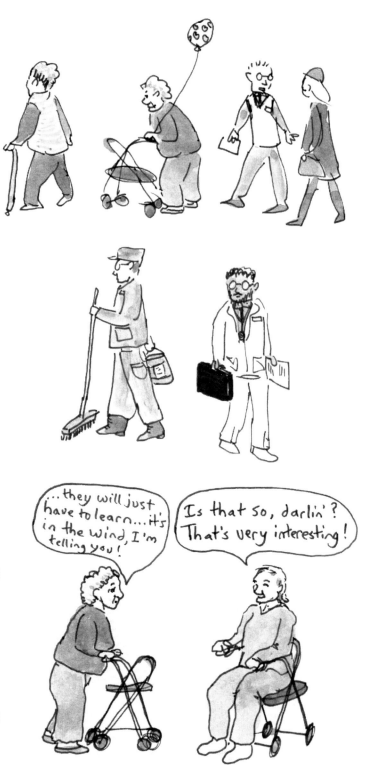

"Get Well" Cards

Plenty of mail came to the house for Aubrey, and I brought him the best of it. Cards and letters from his friends and fans filled up the small bulletin board by his bed, then also a large sheet of paper which I taped to the wardrobe cabinet door. Sometimes these hopeful messages seemed sadly naive, but overall they conveyed undying affection.

Many cards also held donations, which I deposited into his bank account. His fee for room and board at Serenity Shores was just about what he received in Social Security Retirement benefits. Without donations from friends he would not have been able to afford much else besides razors. As it was, he enjoyed getting Chinese take-out with his roommate, and was able to pay back Anu and me when we picked up his medicines and grocery requests.

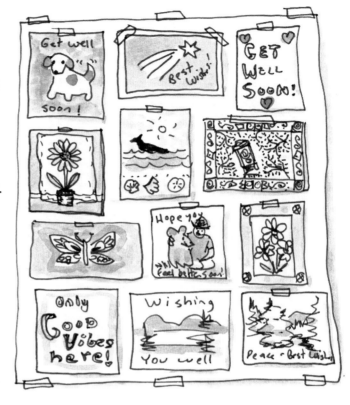

I saved all the envelopes from the get well cards in order to have people's return addresses, knowing the time would come when I would need to write back with thanks and sad news. I honestly didn't have hope in his recovery, nor hope for the prolonging of his life. If his body had been a grape, it seemed as if it were becoming a raisin, and that this process could not be reversed simply by adding special liquid. His spirit, however, seemed fully intact, as large a presence as ever. Whenever I brought him well wishes from people in the outside world, he always said, "Tell them I love them. I love everybody!" He seemed to be more in touch with his heart than I was.

Mostly, I felt tired, serious, and numb. Then, when Steve was about to depart, at the end of the long Presidents Day weekend, I felt a strange thing happening to my face. The veneer of intellectual control cracked open and I burst into tears for the first time since it had all begun. We sat outside in the unseasonably warm sunlight, talked until we were laughing, took a little walk, and went out for coffee. When my balance was restored and I felt able to go on with the day, he (reluctantly) took off down the road, but the intimate warmth of our connection, which had been eclipsed from my consciousness for weeks while I was trying so hard to handle all the changes and chores, was back online.

Angela reassured me that I was not "being negative" to not have hope for Aubrey's recovery. She said that if anyone had their feet on the ground of reality, it was me. His death would come along sooner or later, and someone ought to be preparing. So, among other chores, I continued looking into funeral arrangements and commenced with drafting an obituary.

Couch Surfing

Later that afternoon, Earl and I went shopping for a new couch. At a local furniture store we had fun sitting and bouncing on all the different couches and finally found one we both liked. It was delivered the next day. That week was school vacation, so Earl took charge of breaking in the new couch.

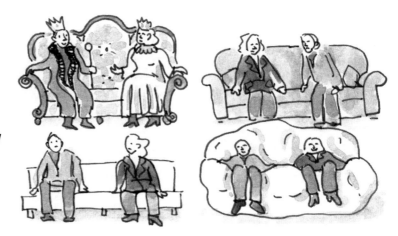

Another cushy part of life was that we still got to have free food deliveries! Aladdin still appeared at the start of every week. I wasn't expecting that, and it felt so kind and supportive. Even though Aubrey wasn't living with us, the people who cooked and delivered the food knew what a challenging time it still was for families going through cancer. The patient's treatment and illness, and not knowing what would change from day to day, was a stress on everyone else. Even with a positive attitude, it was a mental, emotional, and physical workout to dance with having your attention being summoned in service of that person. Some of the somberness and uncertainty were counter-balanced by this physical act of kindness and life affirming care.

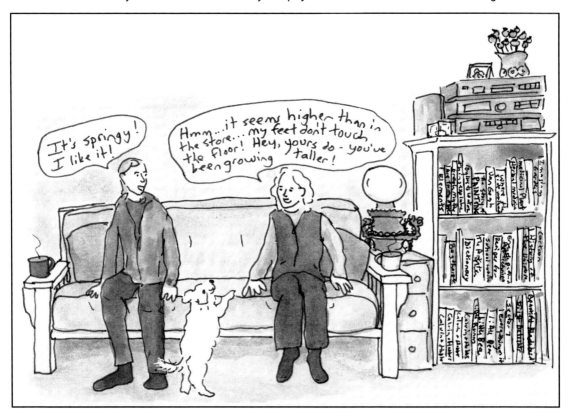

"Persistence Points"

Tuesday, February 21st, in spite of getting a new couch, and knowing I was loved, and having a vacation from school-related chores, I still felt depressed, no appetite, and no oomph to get out of bed. But the dog needed pain pills, and after the vet appointment I was planning to go out for lunch with two friends from out of town. This would be the first time I would sit down with close friends in person and tell them in detail what had been going on this year, and they were dear old friends, so I didn't want to miss the opportunity. So I showed up. It was so worth it! As I shared stories, including how hard it had been to get out of bed that morning, one looked meaningfully at the other and said, "Ah! We need to tell her about Persistence Points!"

Persistence Points was a system they had invented. One was a director at a community theater, the other a Special Ed teacher, so both had training as well as talent in behavior management. This system, however, was for themselves. The deal was, you gave yourself credit for doing hard things, and later could cash those in for rewards. The important part was recognizing the very subjective nature of your persistence. That is, the hard thing might normally be an easy thing, or easy for someone else, but for you, at that time, doing that thing took more than the usual effort. Points earned were equally subjective.

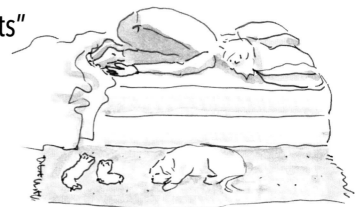

Doing yoga before even getting out of bed... well, child's pose, at least!

You could decide, for example, that getting out of bed today was worth five Persistence Points. Tomorrow it might be easier, only two points, or none. The goal was to value the effort made. I decided I had been wracking up an awful lot of Persistence Points lately, and that the new couch was my reward. It felt so good to talk with them!

That evening, Ella invited Earl and me to her apartment for dinner. She, likewise, lifted us up with her kindness, optimism, and acknowledgement of what we were going through. I explained Persistence Points to her, for she had been earning plenty herself.

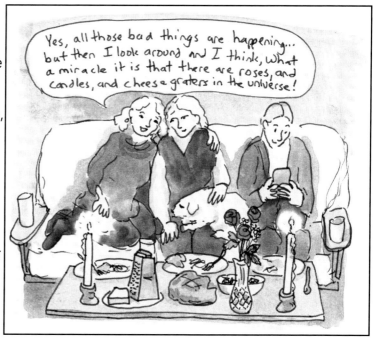

Letters of Evidence

Along with cards, the mail included many bills. Some I had Aubrey write checks for, others I retained, waiting to see what might be retroactively covered whenever the state insurance kicked in. But then a letter came from the state saying that he was denied! We could appeal, if we wished, but the longer it took to complete the application process, the more chance there was that the start date would not cover bills from when the meltdown started in January.

One reason for the denial was that he'd missed a required phone interview. It was on a morning when he was with Anu, on the way to an appointment. The letter telling him to be ready for it had been sent to his post office box, but by the time it got forwarded to my house the date for the interview had passed. Explaining this wasn't a simple matter of calling someone in an office; even hospital personnel, such as doctors, nurses, and social workers, who obviously had much more professional clout than I, would normally be left waiting on-hold for a very long time. With state insurance for myself and Earl, even when I had been given an assigned time to be ready for an interview, I had been left waiting for over an hour until someone there called me. The system seemed lame, if not broken. Not panicking, I reached out to Helpful Hazel, and she kindly offered to make a house call, the afternoon of Thursday, February 23rd. She helped me fill out an appeal, and verified that I needed to track down and submit more documents.

Specifically, there needed to be official letters from all the places Aubrey had worked in the past ten years explaining that he was no longer employed there. Getting them required quite a bit of persistence and thinking like a detective. The hiking camp was closed until summer. The director worked at another job and lived out of state. I used my Facebook connection with a former director who was retired and now a friend of mine, to find out where the new one could be contacted. The YMCA was open, but during that week of winter vacation the person I needed to find was not there until the next week. Likewise, the local schools were closed, so I had to wait for the following week to visit their business office. Addresses for other bus driving gigs Aubrey had listed could be tracked down using the Internet. As for teaching yoga, I typed a letter stating that in the past ten years he had not, to my knowledge, taught anyone yoga for money. Furthermore, even though he had listed "Author" among his professional attributes, as far as I knew there were no recent royalty checks, nor had those ever been a substantial source of income.

It seemed ridiculous to have to go to all the effort of asking so many people to make the effort of writing all those letters (with letterheads, so they would seem official). Wasn't it enough to have a letter from a doctor saying he couldn't drive, and evidence from doctors that he was dying of cancer, and didn't it even count that his current address was a nursing home? The system seemed terribly inefficient.

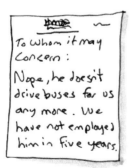

To Whom it may Concern:
Nope, he doesn't drive buses for us any more. We have not employed him in five years.

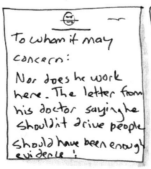

To whom it may concern:
Nor does he work here. The letter from his doctor saying he shouldn't drive people should have been enough evidence!

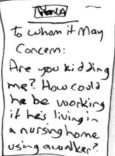

To whom it May Concern:
Are you kidding me? How could he be working if he's living in a nursing home using a walker?

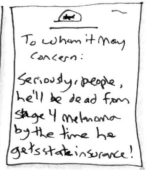

To whom it may concern:
Seriously, people, he'll be dead from stage 4 melnoma by the time he gets state insurance!

Vacation at Home

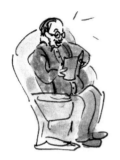 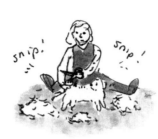 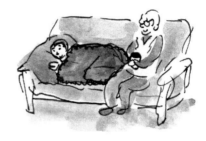

Friday, February 24th, Steve couldn't come for the weekend, but my parents came to read aloud and sip Mumsie water by the fireplace. They admired the new futon couch, and said the room felt renewed. While I was listening, I gave Tucker a trim.

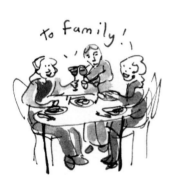 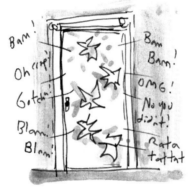 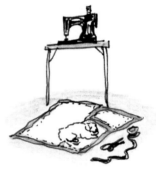

Saturday I actually earned some money doing some cleaning work, then Ella came by for a meal and played video games with Earl while I enjoyed having some creative time alone working on a sewing project.

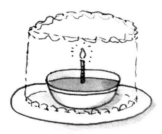 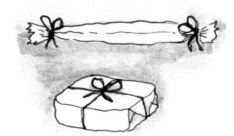

Sunday was Mumsie's birthday, so we all gathered at Mumsie and Grand Pop's house to make merry. She couldn't eat dairy, eggs, flour, cocoa, or sugar, so I baked her an "air cake" and some vegetarian jello made with seaweed. Ella and Earl gave her some hand-dipped beeswax candles and a box of honeycomb.

Travels of Various Kinds

Thank goodness for Serenity Shores and its many services, including on-site doctor visits and van rides to the hospital for special appointments, because Monday, February 27th, Anu and her boyfriend left for a tropical vacation! So as not to paint a picture of her as fancy-free or callous, leaving us in the dust (or snow, as it were), it should be noted that she debated whether to go until the day before the flight, even though she'd been planning it for a year. This allowed Aubrey and me many chances to reassure her that we could manage without her. Aubrey told her she should go. I told her she should go. Aubrey told me to tell her he wanted her to go. And I told Aubrey to tell her that we'd talked and I said it was fine for her to go! At least one of us would be tanned and refreshed. No sense making unnecessary sacrifices!

I had too many other obligations besides Aubrey to even think of "going away" anyway. Ella's dad was the only other person who knew how to take care of the dog's high maintenance needs, and he was out of the country for the rest of the winter. Earl's school vacation was over, so we persisted in getting him to all his music lessons and classes at school.

At home we backed way off on home-schooling, adjusting our expectations from trying to do all subjects and staying on track (in which case we were failing) to instead trying to take better care of ourselves in order to bear the intensity of this novel time. Meeting that goal was more important than any academic subject, although sometimes they were mutually inclusive. For example, we resumed watching documentaries in the evening, taking turns choosing the subject. We'd done that regularly when he was younger, but had stopped as he became more independent. Now, it felt like a cozy thing to look forward to, and it gave us common subjects to discuss: snakes and lizards, black holes and quasars, train rides across continents. Watching these was a mini-vacation from the rest of our waking life.

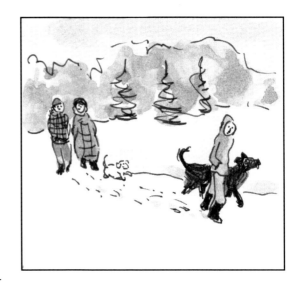

The most important thing for me, as a parent, was staying connected emotionally and in realistic ways. We ate more meals and took more walks together. Sometimes we walked with friends. One had a big dog who seemed to know if Earl was sad. If he was walking alone ahead of us, the dog would trot up and walk beside him. They looked like a mini wolf pack unto themselves. Sometimes we all threw snowballs at each other and slid on the icy crust.

Evening reading of some spiritual literature was a vacation for my mind, giving me temporary relief from worries and fears. Another mind vacation was emailing a couple of friends who were very far away and with whom I was not connected on Facebook, so they hadn't read the medical stories I'd posted. I intentionally kept most of what I was going through out of our conversations in order to safeguard these small islands of communication from being contaminated; it was so refreshing and enjoyable to discuss other things, such as their work and travels abroad.

In an odd way, it seemed as if Aubrey himself were away on a journey; the man we went to see at the nursing home was almost a different person. It felt as if we were just waiting for the real one to return some day. And when he was writing, he seemed to be somewhere far away, in his own imagination.

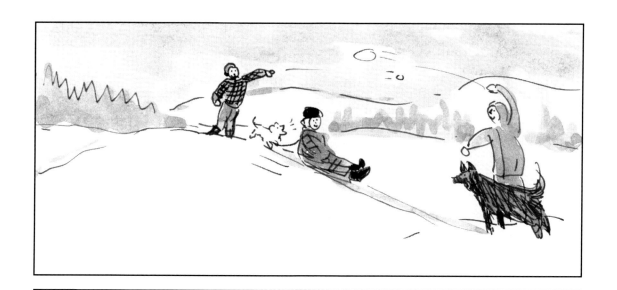

Facebook post Wednesday, March 1, 2017

How am I feeling? Adapting to changes in family life. It's been two months since my son's dad, Aubrey, has been able to meet for their mid-day dog walk (between Aubrey's morning and afternoon bus runs.) It is starting to sink in that, for all practical purposes, I am solo parenting at all times now. I was already used to being Head of Household for most of the years of parenting both of my children, but I had also been accustomed to Aubrey's daily presence in our son's life.

During the past two months I've become accustomed to visiting the newcomer in our midst: this wizened elderly man whose face is contorted by tumors, who is mostly sleeping, who now lives in a nursing home.

But in the back of my mind there has still been an expectation that DAD—the person who is super fit and hikes mountains and does yoga twice a day and eats a simple healthy vegetarian diet (for the most part of the past three decades), who was never even sick with a cold or flu, who we thought was one of the healthiest people we knew—I keep wondering when THIS guy will show up, to tap politely at the back door as he always did, when he returns from wherever he's been off to. (Maybe a spontaneous writer's research trip to New Orleans? Maybe a road trip, or a vision quest along the Appalachian Trail?)

Well, he did CALL me this morning—the man whose sonorous, deep, endearing voice still sounds as healthy as ever—with the good news that tomorrow, while he is at the hospital, having his second immunotherapy infusion, his belongings will be moved from behind the dingy curtained end of a shared room with no view, into a single room with a view of the water.

We'll go visit him there.

5.

The Plot Thickens

Grand Pops Takes the Lead

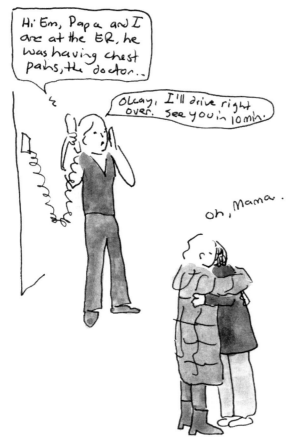

Facebook post Thursday, March 2 at 11:19am

When it rains it pours. So now my dad is about to get a lift in the Life Flight helicopter from our small-town hospital to the big one in the city, for emergency heart surgery. I'm reorganizing my day, trying to line up transportation for my son to and from his lessons, planning for when to drive my mom up to MCMC, in the middle of waiting for call backs from my mom and dad and their neighbors, when a f'ing telemarketer calls me and says in a chirpy voice, "Why, you're as hard to reach as my children!" I give her a hell of a response, rapidly explaining about all the Truly Important Calls I am waiting for! Well, I'm not on THAT call-list any more! She couldn't break script so she ended by saying, "Have a Great Day!" My first thought on hearing about my dad was: at least I already know my way around MCMC: where to park, which elevator, and what floor the cardiology unit is on. Now to go upstairs and tell my son.

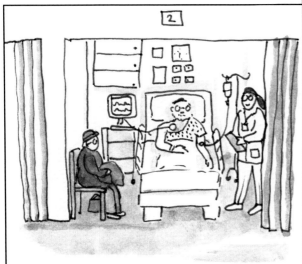

Rational action-based response, activate!

I found my parents in now familiar bay two at the ER, my mom hugging his coat, my dad in a skimpy gown with pastel stripes, shoulder hem unsnapped for access to chest, mobile monitor showing heart beat, blood pressure, and respiration as bright lines with peaks and valleys. He had severe chest pain, was propped up in bed, able to talk and understand, while getting an IV of nitroglycerin. All the doctors and nurses were familiar, so even though it was a serious situation I smiled to see them.

The weather outside was stormy, with dark clouds and strong gusts of wind bearing sleet and rain. Not a safe time for a helicopter ride; besides, he was too fragile to transport, so we waited. Eventually an ambulance was summoned, and my mom rode with him to MCMC. I drove to their house, picked up things they needed, and drove up to meet them. I have no idea what Earl did all day except that I left him in the company of Ella.

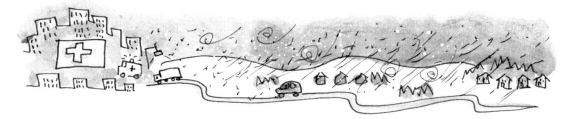

Blood enzymes revealed it was a heart attack, but in tissue with tiny capilaries too small to operate on. When it was clear that there was not going to be surgery, and nothing to decide for the time being, just keeping him overnight for observation, my mom decided she'd catch a ride home with me, feed their cat, make the kind of food she could eat, and get a good night's sleep in her own bed. So home we went through the dark.

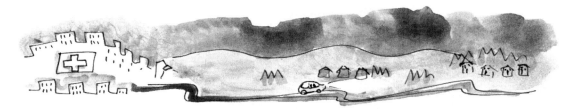

Friday, March 3rd, I picked her up so early that Earl was still asleep, and we returned to MCMC.

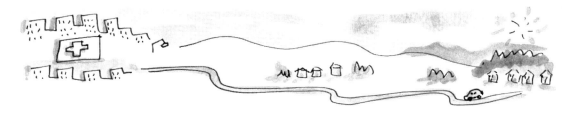

We waited in various lounges while my dad had various procedures and eventually he was given the green light to be discharged. So I drove them home. No need for a neighbor to cat-sit, after all. Ella must have taken Earl to his classes and given him breakfast and lunch. I made dinner, and brought a plate to Aubrey.

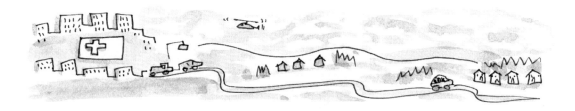

Hurry up and Wait

The thing about a medical emergency is that it renders everything else less important. There is a certain kind of freedom that comes from being given the excuse to drop everything else and attend to the emergency. Time seems to stop. No, not stop so much as to have a gap between past and future, where the present moment expands into an eternity of waiting. At first there may be a feeling of being wrenched away from normal, but there is a certain excitement of being summoned into the unknown.

The initiated come to realize that it is always a good idea to bring along a book. Even when the plot in real life becomes a question of life or death, for characters not on the gurney the role is often "hurry up and wait." Life may offer you gallons more "free time" to sit around and read than you have ever allowed yourself to claim before. Page by page, chapter by chapter, you may find yourself entwining the plot of your loved one's crisis with the romance of some novel's main character, forever hot-wiring these disparate story lines.

With my dad's situation, there was no capacity for me to plan or control anything in the medical realm. I was just living in the moment, going through the motions, doing what I was told to do, or waiting to find out what would happen next, like standing on a beach watching waves. It felt placid. To react with dramatic emotions, to argue with reality by claiming "such and such shouldn't be happening" wouldn't have been wrong, but it would have taken more energy than I had to spend. Coasting along in neutral was the most efficient way to be. There was an ironic sense of ease regarding the familiarity of the places, procedures, and parking lots, as if I were being given an opportunity to put my recent training into practice. Also, prayerfulness was an easy default by now: not praying for certain outcomes for certain people, just asking and listening for guidance and then following it where it led.

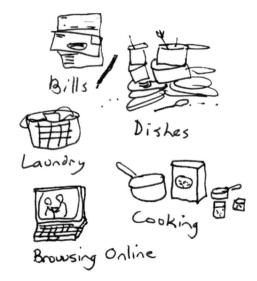

Things Not as Important as Going to the ER

My parents, likewise, were calm, focusing on the practical realities and how to accomplish whatever was within their capability. None of us expressed intense emotions; not that there's anything wrong with that. Our caring was demonstrated by practical actions, rather than emotional words and tears.

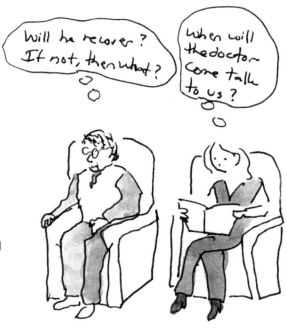

Life (and Death) on the Farm

While my mother and I were traveling between our homes and the hospital, she described how it was for her to take care of her parents at the end of their lives. They were our closest neighbors, living in the house next door, way out in the country, an hour from the city where my dad worked. As my grandparents became infirm it was my mother who played nurse. There was no Hospice in our area back then. She administered shots of morphine for pain control, changed oxygen tanks and dressings on abscesses, and did all the cooking and laundry as well.

I remember walking the foot path between our homes carrying trays of food, and doing chores at their house: stacking firewood, vacuuming, dusting, watering plants, and putting seeds in the bird feeder. Back then my mother spared me the gory details of all that she witnessed and did to help them. But I felt that whatever she was doing for them was as normal as her milking the goats, blanching beans, and putting up applesauce. There was never any sense of drama. Death seemed like a normal part of life. Elderly people becoming bedridden, unable to garden or walk dogs or bake their own bread, was as normal as corn shocks drying in the field, a limb dying on an apple tree, or the barn roof needing shingles. Some problems could be fixed, some couldn't. A person's right relationship to all of this was simply to do the next thing that could be done.

My grandfather died first, the fall I started seventh grade. (By then he was in the hospital.) When my grandmother came home from the hospital that day she canned peaches. That was the next thing that needed doing; the peaches were ripe. ("Waste not, want not." "Make hay while the sun shines." "If you don't have something nice to say, don't say anything at all.") Six years later, my grandmother died in bed at home the day before my high school graduation. The following day my mom (who must have been a sleep-walking zombie by then) put on a graduation party at our house, with my sister's help.

I can't recall my parents or grandparents crying over the death of a relative–not that they didn't, but if they did, they did it in private. When one of our farm animals or house pets died, however, my mother took it pretty hard. There was a special place on the farm where dogs, cats, chickens, geese, and goats were buried. I wasn't as attached to any of them, so I never felt upset. Then again, the deaths of my grandparents never brought me to tears, either. Perhaps it was their long decline into terrible health that helped mitigate any sorrow I might have had, and if they'd died more suddenly and by surprise that would have been harder to handle. As it was, release from suffering in a body wracked with pain and no longer capable of walking or breathing with ease seemed like a good thing.

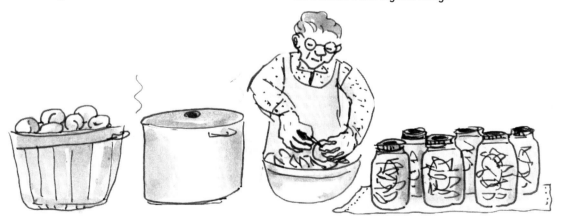

147

Happy Interlude

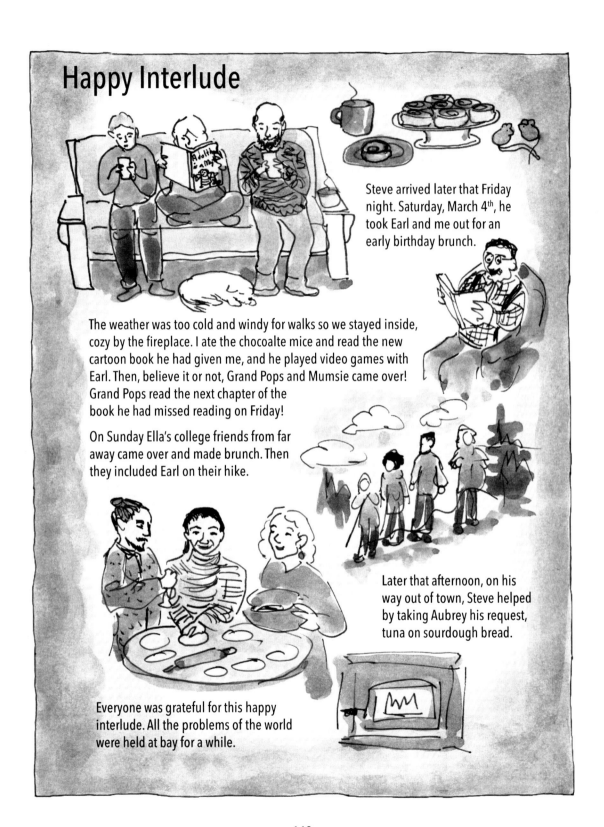

Steve arrived later that Friday night. Saturday, March 4th, he took Earl and me out for an early birthday brunch.

The weather was too cold and windy for walks so we stayed inside, cozy by the fireplace. I ate the chocoalte mice and read the new cartoon book he had given me, and he played video games with Earl. Then, believe it or not, Grand Pops and Mumsie came over! Grand Pops read the next chapter of the book he had missed reading on Friday!

On Sunday Ella's college friends from far away came over and made brunch. Then they included Earl on their hike.

Later that afternoon, on his way out of town, Steve helped by taking Aubrey his request, tuna on sourdough bread.

Everyone was grateful for this happy interlude. All the problems of the world were held at bay for a while.

More of Everything

Monday morning, March 6th, there was another surprise phone call from my parents. They were back in the ER at SBH, had been since early that morning. My dad was having another slow burning heart attack. I knew they were concerned to get their Living Wills redone in our state (another name for Advance Directives). That had been on their to-do list before this new plot twist, so I texted Angela to see if she could meet them in the ER and help them get those forms filled out. It felt comforting to see her again, someone familiar with our other story. By the time it was decided to send my dad up to MCMC again it was dinner time. Since he was stabilized and no big decisions needed to be made until morning, I drove my mom home for the night.

But first, we stopped off at my house, where another jolly party was being held. Everyone sat on the living room floor in front of the fireplace while Tucker the dog made the rounds, inspecting and sniffing at the Chinese dumplings, spring rolls and dipping sauces, the miso soup, green tea, and mochi ball ice cream. This scene conveyed a sense of safety and warmth, a community of wordly people taking care of one another, openly celebrating in spite of the many crises. My mom and I basked in the glow before going back out into the cold wintry night. When I got back home I was very glad to find them all still there, debating and laughing and keeping the fire alive.

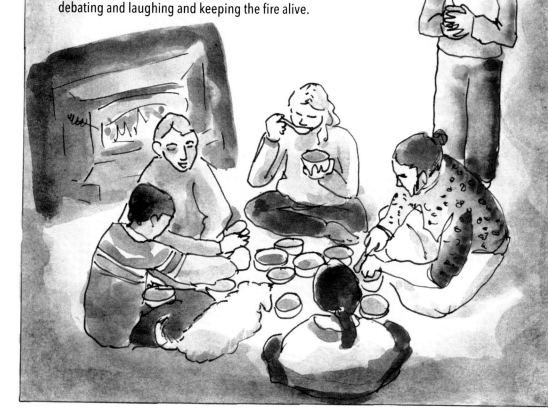

Things to Discuss in the Waiting Room

Tuesday, March 7th, I picked up my mom at the crack of dawn and drove back to MCMC, then drove home through a snow storm in time to get Earl to school and field a food request from Aubrey, who seemed to be holding steady (at least he led me to believe so). Our visits were reduced to these short drop-offs of food, a brief exchange of "How are you?" and the reliable closing remarks, "I love you, here's a hug."

Wednesday, March 8th, after breakfast, I drove up to the city again, bringing my mom some food she could eat since the cafeteria was not an option. The plan was to discharge my dad, but he had a splitting headache and looked very pale. While we all waited for the discharge process to be signed off by everyone, he tried to nap. My mother and I talked in the waiting area of the hospital lobby near the giant potted palms.

<u>Things to Discuss in the Waiting Room</u>

- If they discharge him today, do you feel confident taking care of him at home by yourself?
- Can you guys afford the new super expensive medication that Medicare won't cover?
- Should the other daughter be summoned yet? Here, call her on my phone.
- Will he still be allowed to drive? If not, how often will you be needing rides for groceries?
- What if he dies soon? Could you live where you are on your own?
- Do you know where he hides all the passwords?

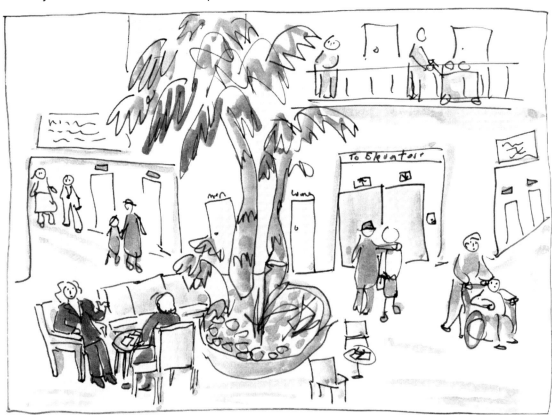

Birthday Blues

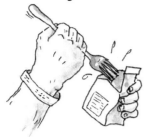

When we visited my dad around lunch time, he was feeling cranky and miserable and having a hard time with his executive functioning and coordination. His fumbled attempts to open a carton of milk led to a violent attack on the carton. He didn't seem in any shape to go home. Much to my mother's and my relief, after nearly three hours of deliberation the doctors decided he was still too fragile to discharge. They also discovered that one of the IV medicines inexplicably had corn in its list of ingredients. This was a known allergen that my dad had explicitly warned everyone–from nurses and doctors to dietitians–to avoid at all costs, because it caused him to have severe headaches! Oh well.

When the nurse brought his lunch tray she asked, "Birthday?" She meant for him to tell her his birth date, while she double checked the numbers on his wrist band, a protocol that happened every time they gave patients food, medicine, or any kind of test.

"Yes! It's my daughter's birthday!" he replied.

After repeating her question and getting the same response, she realized he meant me. "Oh! Congratulations! Twenty-nine, I presume?" she asked, sweetly.

"No, fifty!" I shot back, "I hope I'm at least half way done with this crazy life!" I guess the tension was infectious. However, our visit ended on a more cheerful note, with hugs, kisses, a birthday card and check, and hopes for the best for everyone.

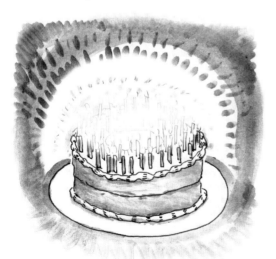

Facebook post Wednesday, March 8

Just home from the big hospital, not bringing my dad home after all. He's been there since Monday. Monday, Tuesday, and Wednesday this week I've logged in many hours in transit to visit my folks at our small-town hospital's ER, ICU, and then in the cardiac unit at MCMC. Last week's episode was indeed a kind of heart attack, as was this Monday's episode. Not the dramatic kind of sudden attack we think of people pantomiming, more of a long slow burn that leaves enzyme markers indicating the level of damage to heart tissues. There is no clear path of what to do about it going forward, but my folks report there are good doctors who give them way more time and attention than anywhere else they have lived. Now I'm gonna go party with my dear children whenever they let me come downstairs to see what they have been working on!

Ella and Earl had baked me a truly fabulous birthday cake, with fancy piped-on lemon-lavender frosting. There were so many candles the frosting was melting! It was a sight to behold! After cake they took me out to dinner. You know what they say: "Life is uncertain, so eat dessert first!"

Childhood's End?

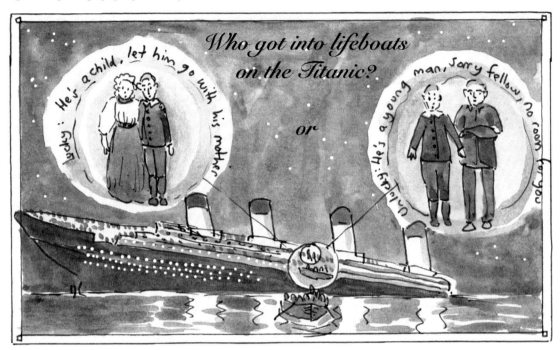

My dad's infirmity caused me to contemplate the possibility of his death, and the difference between the death of one's dad when one is fifty, fifteen, or thirteen. I would miss him, but I had decades of memories, and would be able to help my mother with anything as an equal adult. Aubrey had been fifteen when his father died, and the message he got, whether it was spoken by others, implied, or self-generated was, "You are now the man of the family. Take care of your mother and little brother." (That heavy trip was not without some fallout.)

The fate of his son, two years younger, was more ambiguous. Earl could be seen as an older child or as a young man, depending on where he lived, what society he was in, and what period of history it was. Taking all that into account, it was apparent that life was handing him the grace of being taken care of as a child, somewhat sheltered from responsibilities, but also dealing him the loss of his dad by his side to guide him during his transition into adulthood. A future "father figure" might appear, but Earl would only ever have thirteen years with his own dad.

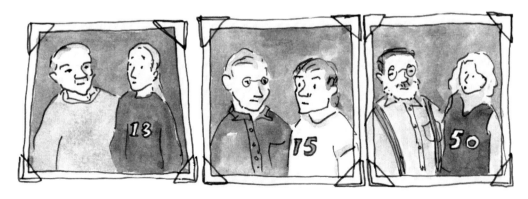

Childhood Revisited

During each of my dad's heart attacks more heart tissue died. He could take the expensive new medicine the cardiologist prescribed (yet Medicare wouldn't cover), and carry around a bottle of nitroglycerin pills to pop at the onset of any symptoms of further heart attacks, but there was no surgical solution in sight. My uncertainty of how much time he had left triggered a cascade of childhood memories and somber ruminations. Thursday, March 9th, he was able to be discharged. I transported my folks to their house, then headed home to mine.

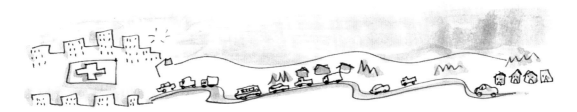

Over the weekend Rhia came to visit her dad and look for jobs in the area. Sunday, March 12th, she stopped by the house just as I was about to leave for an appointment. After quick hugs and how are yous I asked her if she'd like to hang out with Earl for a bit. There happened to be a photo album out on the table that we'd just found in a closet. So she sat downstairs on the new couch with her little brother and they looked at the album together: an ordinary family scene, but this was their first time doing a thing together, just the two of them, ever! She found photos of herself and Ella when we briefly lived as a blended family, and they found photos of themselves with their dad. As they reminisced, they realized that they shared some common happy memories of "Dad time." The interesting thing was, these events had happened several years apart!

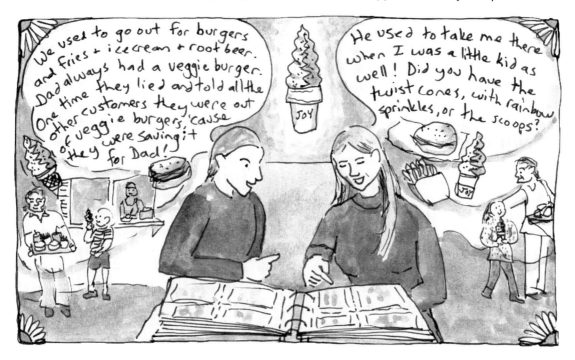

Dad's Salad

They both knew about "Dad Salad," which was his stock contribution to every potluck supper and special family dinner that ever was. Everyone loved it! He always served it in a wide flat ceremic bowl that had large flowers on it.

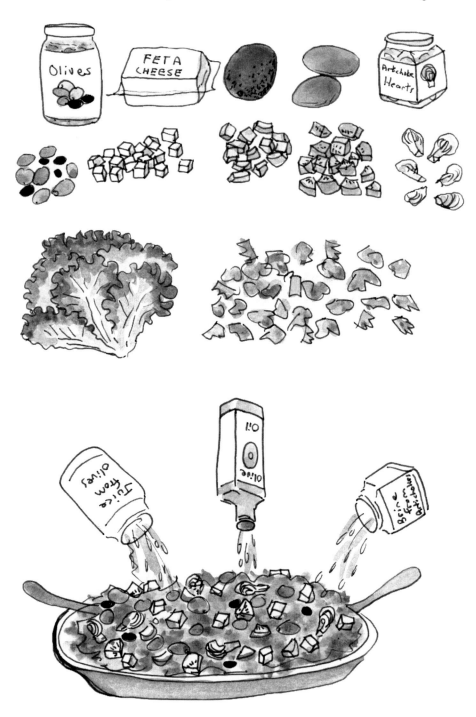

Monday, March 13th, Aubrey showed me a video about a special cancer-fighting salad. He'd been telling me about this salad for several days. His personal goal for daily nutrition was to drink a smoothie, eat a small lunch, and have this cancer-fighting salad as dinner. He'd asked The Cook if he could make the salad for him, and The Cook offered to provide some of the ingredients, such as spinach and broccoli.

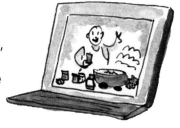

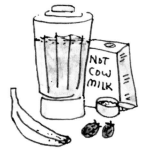

After watching the video I went to the store and bought all the other ingredients. They all seemed healthy, but I was doubtful that they would help him get better at this point, and with open sores in his mouth I doubted that eating such things as apple cider vinegar and red pepper flakes would be a "healing experience." Fulfilling his request was what really mattered.

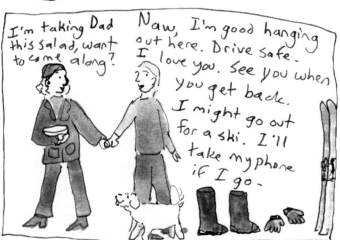

I'm taking Dad this salad, want to come along?

Naw, I'm good hanging out here. Drive safe. I love you. See you when you get back. I might go out for a ski. I'll take my phone if I go.

When I brought him these ingredients the next day he was not interested to eat anything. When I showed him the jar of vinegar and olive oil, and the shaker bottle with all the spices, he said it all seemed overwhelming. His appetite had been getting weaker since the second immunotherapy infusion. As I could see from the weekly charts he was still keeping, he'd been losing weight for the past two weeks, about half a pound per day.

His face looked gaunt and famished. There were little cups of juice and bowls of fruit sitting in his windowsill to get warm, since he didn't like to eat or drink cold food. But he wasn't remembering to eat or drink them before they spoiled. I kept throwing them away because no one else seemed to notice. His mini fridge was getting full of food that was past its due date, including sandwiches he'd requested from home. The idea of certain foods was still appealing, but consuming them was not. He explained

that he didn't feel like eating because it took so much time and effort which got in the way of his writing time.

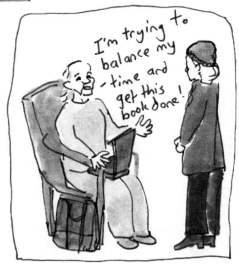

I'm trying to balance my time and get this book done!

Into the Depths

In early January, when the impact of Aubrey's cancer was a new influence in our lives, there had been a sense of having a "normal life" that was being impacted by a novel event.

By mid March, the novelty had morphed into a surrounding and penetrating influence, affecting every moment of daily life. It was like the strong smell of wood smoke in the air which you can't avoid smelling, or persistent sounds that you can't turn off. Even though he wasn't living with us, the unstoppable decaying of his physical form and the inevitability of his death invoked a unique atmosphere that permeated daily life no matter what we were doing, confronting us with the blunt reality of the inevitability of death, the ending of a body's viability to function in the world. We contemplated his mortality and our own, and how little control we had over any of it.

The relentlessness of this confrontation of mortality wasn't something I would have consciously sought or wished for, but I recognized it as a gift, a kind of sacred time. It took me beyond the theoretical and intellectual contemplation of death and dying, into profound depths of feeling and awareness that I didn't even know existed. As with the unique period of life in the days after giving birth, it was an experience that could not be otherwise manufactured; only the reality of the unique situation could bring on these feelings. It was an initiation experience after which one goes through life permanently changed.

Aubrey and I never discussed his dying directly. Part of "being in the pit" with him was "meeting him where he was at" and not forcing that conversation. The closest I came was telling him of a dream I had in which he set his finished manuscript on my kitchen table, then dissolved, leaving only a pile of clothing on the floor.

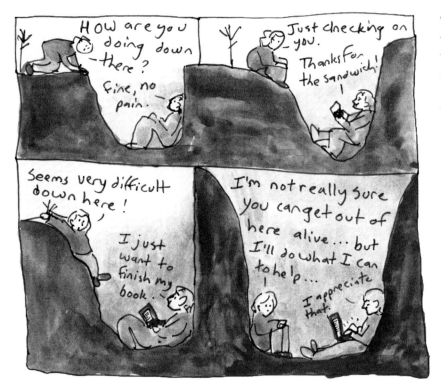

While one is down in this pit, abiding with the loved one who is dying, that's when any kind of support from the community is really awesome. I was happily surprised to get a package in the mail from a mystery person, containing two chocolate bars and a note: "I know this doesn't fix anything but at least it's a sweet distraction for a moment's time." That was really nice, and it did bring some cheer!

Difficult Discussions about Death and Decay

Tuesday, March 14th, the day of the uneaten salad, was a snow day off from school, so I stayed for a longer visit than usual with Aubrey. Anu was still away, and Rhia was back at work, and it seemed important for one of us to have a longer check-in with him. Rhia had told me over the weekend that he seemed to have a hard time following conversations. As well as losing his appetite, he'd also stopped shaving. He hadn't showered in a week and had been wearing the same clothing all week. His bedroom smelled rank. If he were a dog or cat I'd be guessing he was in his final days: when a mammal stops grooming it usually means something is very wrong inside.

While I was visiting him the nurses stopped in briefly. Each time, he'd tell them he was fine and didn't need anything. He wasn't interested in being helped. Just undisturbed time to write, thank you very much. When I asked him about shaving and bathing he said he'd get to it. I knew from past experience that when he felt pressured to do a thing he seemed to resist doing it even more, so I tried to pussy-foot around it and not come across as pushy. However, I also recognized that in brief conversational exchanges with the nurses one might make the assumption that he was still able to make clear choices and be fairly independent, but from knowing him more deeply, I could tell that he was slipping.

There was also a problem with pills. Soon after he'd moved to Serenity Shores, he'd gotten permission to take his morning pills on his own. However, lately, he confided, he was becoming so deeply lost in thought about his writing that he would forget to take his morning pills until long past the appointed hour. Now that I was aware of this he agreed we should ask the nurses for more help with that.

On my way out of the building I had a chat with The Matron, sharing my concerns about the smells and Aubrey's need for more support with shaving and bathing. She was aware that it was becoming more difficult for him to take care of himself, but she explained that he was also reticent to receive assistance and he kept telling everyone that he could take care of such things himself, thank you very much. I laughed in sympathy, and told her I was familiar with that dynamic. Oh, the indignities of being a highly independent person facing one's physical decline!

Early the next morning, Wednesday, March 15th, the ringing phone woke me up. It was The Matron, reporting that Aubrey was being sent to Small Brick Hospital by ambulance. There were signs of internal bleeding and the threat of heart failure. I quickly dressed, told Earl where I was going, and drove to the ER.

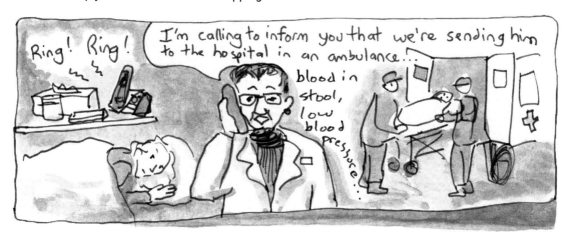

When they asked if he'd seen black stool (from blood) before that morning he explained, "No. It was red, so I figured that was fresh healthy blood." He was dehydrated from massive blood loss and his blood pressure was critically low. A nurse checked his blood glucose and it was also critically low. His thinking could have easily become compromised from low blood sugar, never mind all the rest! They gave him many things to help, including a saline drip and three blood transfusions. He spent the night in intensive care.

The next morning, Thursday, March 16th, he looked rosy cheeked and bright eyed due to all those interventions. He was feeling so chipper that he couldn't fathom why he was being kept in the hospital, and claimed that everyone was overreacting! I was in the room when they explained everything to him, and could tell he wasn't following all of it. He would stare blankly past us, and make little motions and sounds that could be interpreted as signs of active listening, but those were the "uh huh" sounds one makes when one is distracted and just faking that one is listening. I knew he was not following all the explanations. For weeks already I had been adjusting how I talked to him to be more simplified. As much as I could, I stayed nearby to be part of those medical discussions and "translate" for him.

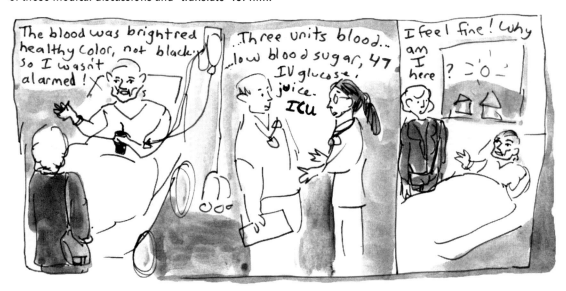

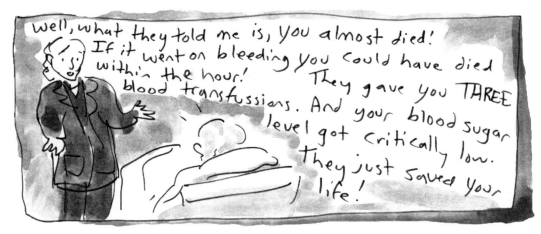

On the day he was admitted, and during the next two days, I met with Angela, the visiting oncologist, and other doctors who were on-duty at different times. They each took time to explain and discuss everything with me. It was common for patients with melanoma to die from internal bleeding. They couldn't offer an estimate of how much time he might have left, but they said it could be very close to the end. Aubrey viewed the blood transfusions as a "cure" because he felt so much livelier, but the doctors explained that he was not going to recover, that his bodily systems were starting to fail, and that there would be greater decline in the days to come. Low appetite was a common side effect of immunotherapy, and his rapid weight loss was also due to the cancer: it was digesting his own tissues to fund itself! He probably had bleeding in the digestive tract. They said they could do an invasive and painful procedure by putting a scope down his throat to check for ulcers in his stomach, but that even if they found something there was not much to be done about it. Aubrey agreed to have that procedure, but I quickly intervened. I explained to him that the doctors had to keep telling him everything they *could* offer, but that didn't mean they were *recommending* it, nor that it would improve his health or quality of life. Right away people around us nodded, and when he decided not to have the procedure there was a palpable wave of relief throughout the room.

Through these discussions Aubrey was mostly quiet. He also responded by chanting, "By the light of my heart, I dissolve tumors." He explained that he was healing himself with this mantra, and that true healing is in the mind and that he was using his mind to heal himself. He explained that writing was the most important thing for him to be doing in life because his book was about transformation. He felt the words were encoded with healing vibrations, and that working on the writing connected him with those vibrations. His goal was to finish his novel. Otherwise, he talked in riddles for the better part of his three-day stay: obtuse sentence fragments that sounded like notes taken during a philosophy lecture. At one point he asked me, "Am I making sense to you?"

I answered, "I sense that you are seeing something that I'm not seeing, and that what you are saying is coherent and makes sense to you. But what I'm hearing are a lot of separate thoughts that don't add up–for me."

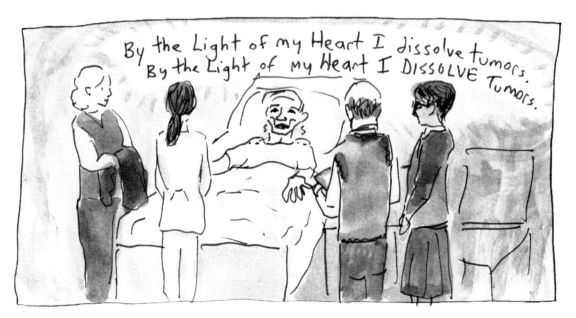

Everyone helping him at the hospital respected his bravery and perseverance, and I think we each caught glimpses of truth in some of the things he was saying. Transformation, on a spiritual and psychological plane, was certainly possible. And sometimes miraculous healing took place on the physical level. One could hope.

But there was also the possibility that death was on its way, and so there were down-to-earth practical matters to face. The biggest issue, which I felt caught in the middle of, was Code 1 versus DNR. It was a consensus on the part of all the medical people, as well as Angela and The Matron, that Aubrey would be better served by changing his status from Code 1 to DNR. What did "Code 1" mean, and why was the "DNR" form so important? As with all the rest of the formal choices and paperwork, I learned about it as I encountered it. At first everyone used technical jargon that left one guessing–unless one had done a Google search and knew what some of the issues were. I had a clue, but I wanted it spelled out clearly in his specific case. Being "Code 1" status meant that he wanted to be kept alive at all costs, with every means possible. That sounded life-affirming to him. If his heart stopped, they'd do CPR. Everyone knows CPR is a good thing, right? As they explained, it depended on the condition of one's body. If he passed out, or stopped breathing, or his heart stopped, all means of resuscitation and artificially extending his life would be employed. If he entered a comatose vegetative state he'd be kept alive with a feeding tube and a ventilator. For a younger, more healthy person, resuscitation (such as after a catastrophic car accident) could buy some time, and with time, some healing or even recovery back to a high quality of life might be possible. But in Aubrey's case, with the cancer so advanced and his organs already so compromised, the actions of resuscitation would absolutely be certain to break bones and damage his heart even more, leaving him in much worse condition, with a lot more pain, than before the resuscitation. What kind of life would he have in such a damaged body? It helped me understand when they explained it in these graphic terms.

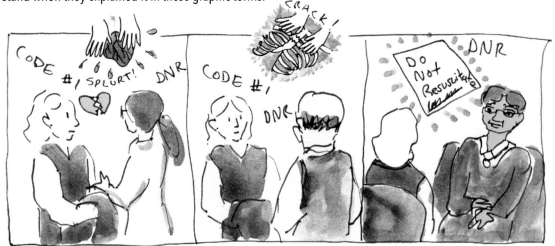

Aubrey's response to these dismal scenarios was to dismiss them. "I don't see that being necessary, it won't come to that." We all tried to explain that because he was choosing to be Code 1 status, if it *did* come to that, those were the actions the nurses and doctors at the hospital (or at Serenity Shores) had to take, by law. Everyone hoped that I might somehow help him come to grips with his situation, get him to change his mind, and sign the DNR, for his own sake. But when I tried to talk to him he wouldn't engage. When a nurse came in he said to her (about me), "When she looks at me, she sees death." He equated the DNR with giving up.

On the third morning, Friday, March 17th, he was still fragile enough that the plan was to keep him in the ICU. If he survived the weekend, a "palliative care team" meeting was being planned for Monday, March 20th.

Earl was going away on a home-school adventure that weekend, to (hopefully) have fun with several other families, so it was important to let him know how close his dad might be to the end. But his dad's appearance had changed so much since Earl had last seen him that I thought it would be a shock. So I contacted Aladdin, and took him up on his earlier offer. To my relief he was available to come over, meet at the house with Earl, and explain how bodies can change at the end of life, especially under the influence of cancer. He gave Earl time to talk and ask questions, then they went to the ICU together. Later Earl told me it went well.

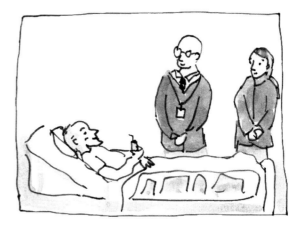

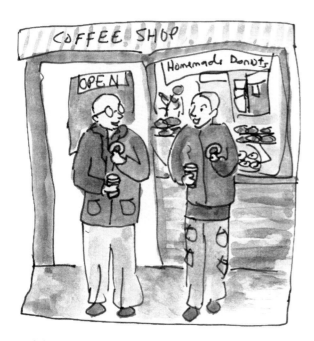

While they were hanging out, I had talks with all the doctors, Angela, and Aubrey. The visiting oncologist made a strong recommendation to discontinue immunotherapy, explaining that it was not helping, and might even be causing some of the internal bleeding. When he asked Aubrey if he wanted to "never go back" to see his oncologist, Aubrey was concerned by the word "never" and wanted to connect at least one more time for closure, and keep the option open to continue immunotherapy later if his bleeding stopped and he felt up for it. The next infusion was supposed to be in a week, but that was discouraged because it could lead to further hemorrhaging. I suggested an appointment be made for the end of the month so he could meet with his oncologist one more time, for closure. He liked that idea, so an appointment was made for March 30th.

He didn't like being stuck in the hospital. He complained about being stuck in a hospital bed with all those IV tubes stuck in his arm. He just wanted to go home to his room at Serenity Shores, work on his book, and have privacy to focus on his healing meditations. So, all together, we hashed out a new plan. The plan we all agreed to–Aubrey, me, the doctor on duty, and a nurse as a witness who double-checked with him at discharge–was to discontinue all forms of treatment and let him do his spiritual healing work free from chemicals. Other than a sleep aid and an anti-anxiety medication (if he wanted some), he would stop taking all prescriptions and stop the immunotherapy. But he still didn't want to sign the DNR.

Just before noon, the cut-off time when a weekend stay would have been inevitable, he was given the option to be discharged. He was very pleased. When a doctor and nurse checked with him again about the plan he enthusiastically agreed. Everyone reassured him that his choice to go back to his room, write, and do his healing meditations was valid and that we all stood behind him. Everyone at the hospital was on the same page.

Since there was no medical emergency or appointment to get to, neither the ambulance nor the van from the nursing home was an option. He needed a family member or friend to drive him back, so I did. As we were riding together the car filled up with a smell like rotting meat.

When The Matron checked with him again, to be sure he understood the new plan, he acknowledged that he understood, and reasserted what he wanted: to purify his body, stop putting chemicals into it, and do spiritual healing, "from the light of his heart."

One more task had to be completed before I could relax for the weekend. All the other home-school parents who would be in charge of Earl needed to be informed that it was possible that his dad might not make it through the weekend. They needed to be ready to console him and bring him home right away, if necessary. As I was editing that email letter in an effort to make it sound less dramatic, I laughed out loud. The fact was, the situation *was* dramatic! "Please take note: the kid's dad might die while he's away this weekend."

Or he might not. It wasn't certain enough to cancel the fun. Earl really needed some fun, for a change! As did I. Good thing my boyfriend wasn't adverse to joining me in the midst of all this focus on death and decay! He was a good sport, listening to my tales from the past two weeks, acting appropriately impressed, offering sympathy and unflagging good humor.

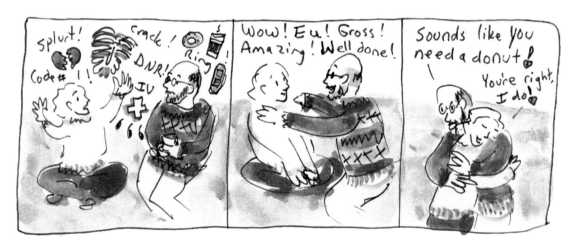

Late that same night, delayed a day by a blizzard, Anu and her boyfriend finally made it home.
My sister arrived at our parents' house.
She brought Aubrey a pair of hand-knitted socks, which he wore every day for the rest of his life.
Further difficult discussions about death, decay, and end-of-life choices took place over the weekend.
Earl had a really fun time away with his friends.
Steve and I really did get donuts, and they were good.

A Room with a View

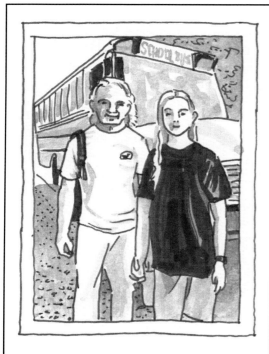

Support a Community Member in Need

~~~~

Update 3/18/17
Dear friends and community members,

Here is the view from Aubrey's new room at Serenity Shores. He can see the water from his windows. There was a bald eagle flying nearby when we visited today.

I talked with one of the nurses and she said all the team there really appreciates him for his good nature, patience, and kindness. She was glad to be providing a private room for him and said they all wanted to do anything they could to make his stay comfortable.

Thank you all for your donations, cards, and love. Aubrey sends love to you.

With all the goings on regarding my dad and Aubrey in March, I'd gotten behind on posting updates. (They aren't required, but are encouraged if you're doing an online fundraiser.) He had moved to his new room on the same day as my dad's first heart attack, the same day as the second immunotherapy infusion. By Saturday, March 18th, when I posted this update, many things had changed besides his view, but it didn't seem appropriate to share most of that at the time. I kept the focus on the positive, and shared a photo of the view of stead of a mugshot of the man because he looked so startlingly different. He'd never liked having his photo taken, anyway, and it certainly wasn't the time to pressure him to pose. Besides, he was trying to focus on his work.

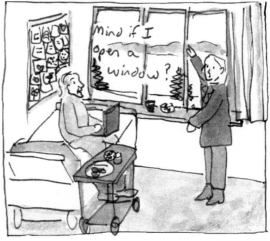

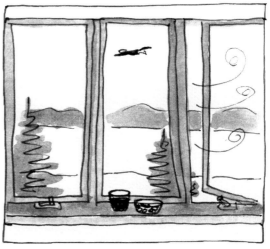

A Boring Week

A whole week went by without anyone going to the hospital! Anu was back to accompany Aubrey to appointments. So I focused more on Earl, home-schooling, dog walks, cleaning work, talking with friends, and updating my "Log of Health and Events Regarding Aubrey Bart." This wasn't a required task, but it seemed important. It could be shared with Anu and Rhia, and perhaps some day Earl would want to know more about his dad's last days. In any case, writing was my main way of processing. The only notable event between Sunday, March 19th and Sunday, March 26th was described by The Matron. She observed that Aubrey had "turned the corner: from denial to anger" (in the stages of death and dying) and was taking it out on the nurses. We all suspected that he was also feeling pain, but if he was, he denied it.

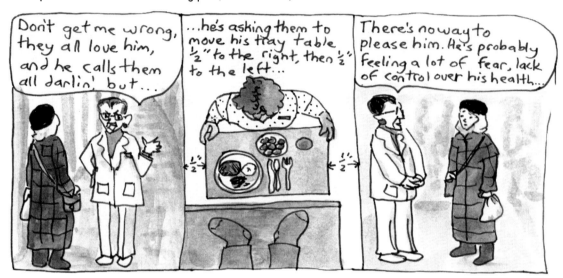

I visited almost daily, sometimes twice a day, often bringing food that he had asked for, but he mostly didn't eat it. One day he asked for a tuna sandwich. It was sitting in the same spot two days later. He didn't eat most food The Cook sent either. He sent it back or threw it away. He threw away most of the carbohydrate rich foods, such as toast, just eating the eggs the kitchen sent him for breakfast.

One day he told me the only solid food he had interest in were steamed greens. I brought bags of organic greens to the kitchen because he said they had agreed to cook them for him. But when I took the greens to the kitchen, The Cook had a different story. They could not prepare food that was brought in from the outside, unless it was a delivery from their official food service. It was against the institutional safety regulations.

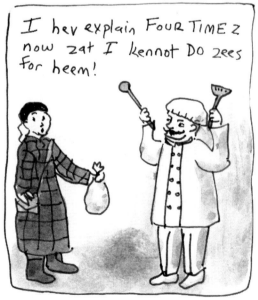

Facebook post #1 Thursday, March 23

A week ago, Wednesday, March 15, my son's dad Aubrey was back in the hospital. Three blood transfusions and other interventions stabilized him enough to return last Friday to his nice quiet private room-with-a-view at the nursing home. He's back to working on his novel with all the attention of a professional writer.

There is the tension of feeling "on call" because the phone might ring at 8 am, or 8 pm, and I have been ready to respond with listening, explaining, writing, driving, shopping, and cooking what is desired. I have not minded being called by nurses and residential care directors for updates on his health status, and have truly enjoyed talking in person to nurses and doctors at the hospital. Honestly, it is easier for me, and more interesting, when there is some novel action, some development in the plot, some new information to be learned. I find it easier to feel strong, calm, engaged, alert, and present in the ICU than in my house, where everything is pretending to look cheerful and stable, trying to carry on with "normal" daily life—if that is even a thing anymore.

Time seems very slow as I do boring household tasks such as folding laundry, vacuuming, boiling noodles, and chopping vegetables. Finally I'm bored enough to tackle the pile of envelopes: the bill for over a thousand for the ambulance, thousands from the nursing home, many thousands more from two hospitals and several labs. They cover the living room floor until I file each receipt and put a note in each return envelope with the new insurance number, hoping some debt can be absorbed.

Having finished that chore, nothing else seems as important or demanding. But there's not enough attention left for having a creative appetite. No projects appeal, no books call to be read. Some animal instinct inside me recommends "taking it easy" whenever I can, in case things get wild again without warning. The plot lines of Aubrey and my dad's health crises are coloring everything this year. I'm trying to remember that things won't always be this way, but it's easy to see impermanence and fragility everywhere.

Facebook post #2 Thursday, March 23

My attention span is too short for novels or nonfiction texts, but I'm enjoying some graphic memoirs such as *Can't We Talk About Something More Pleasant?* by cartoonist Roz Chast. I'd recommend it as a fun way to broach the topic of end-of-life care with those you may end up caring for. Or at least it's an entertaining book if you're in need of a way to laugh about the anxiety, frustration, stress, responsibilities, and lack of control you're having or may have in such a situation. Read it and laugh, read it and weep, read it and rage about the limitations of health care, insurance, and elder care in the USA. It also gives an honest portrait of the challenges of parent-child relationships as everyone gets older.

Other Visitors

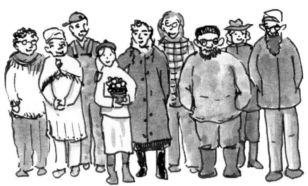

By the fourth week of March the weather was quite mild some days, and the air had that melty earthy smell of early spring. Aubrey worked on his computer every morning, so I tried to visit mostly in the afternoons. His energy continued to go downhill, so I kept visits short. He usually sat quietly, leaving the talking to me. He wasn't energized enough to say much or respond much when talked to. He didn't have energy for personal grooming. He hadn't bathed or changed his clothes since coming home from the hospital.

When Earl got back from the fun weekend away, he came along for a visit. Fortunately, Aubrey was able to rally his the attention and enthusiasm to hear about Earl's adventures. Ella came along with us that day. She showed him pictures she'd taken of Earl, and they all shared some laughs.

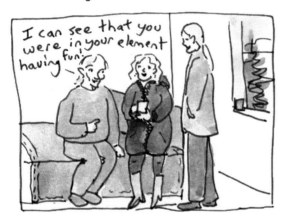

Earl could tell his dad still wasn't ready to accept that he was dying, so they talked about other things: school, skiing, the eagle sitting in the tree near the open window. Later I asked Earl how he was doing. He explained he was aware his dad could die at any time, but it was no longer a shocking idea. He explained that he'd already said all the things he needed to get off his chest and share, for closure, back in January, in the ER. Not being melodramatic, simply candid, he said the dad he'd been attached to already seemed to have died.

I could relate to that. My relationship with my ex had passed through many phases. In the current phase, most of my attention was taken up by the mundane business and medical side of things. He called upon me for help with food and finances. It was easy to forget that there was more to the story, and more going on in the life of the patient. Fortunately, we family members weren't the only people looking after him. From the guest book at the front desk in the lobby, it was apparent that plenty of other people were visiting him as well. Nurse Bea came often to do Reiki. The Turbanator and The Farmer visited frequently. Carpenter Man made visits during the early hours of the morning several times a week. Once in a while our paths crossed in the hallway, as if it were a shift change at work. Fans and friends from out of town also came visiting, some calling my house first, but most contacting Aubrey directly. He had friends from many eras of his life, and a diverse spiritual community as a source of comfort and support.

From the sign-in and sign-out times in the guest book, it was apparent that some people were spending way more time with him than Earl and I were. I hoped they weren't wearing him out and taking away his writing time. And I felt a bit envious, imagining him spending "quality time" with them as friends. But mostly I felt grateful that there were other people offering him their care and attention.

Turning the Corner

All day Monday, March 27th, I felt a sense of anticipation, just waiting for the phone to ring.

Early the next morning, the phone woke me up, and again it was The Matron. She explained that she needed to send Aubrey to Small Brick Hospital by ambulance because his blood pressure was very low, there were new signs of internal bleeding, but he was resisting transport, wouldn't shut off his computer, said he just wanted to keep writing. "But he's Code 1, so we have to send him." Could I come over and help? We talked briefly about what Code 1 implied, and she almost pleaded with me to help him see the light. If any of her nurses found him passed out, they'd have to do CPR, and he was so fragile it would certainly break his ribs, and this would traumatize them and not end up making him better, just leave him broken–if he even survived it. I said I'd try again to talk him into it. By the time I was dressed she called back. He had allowed them to put him on the gurney and wheel him out to the ambulance, so I drove right to the hospital instead.

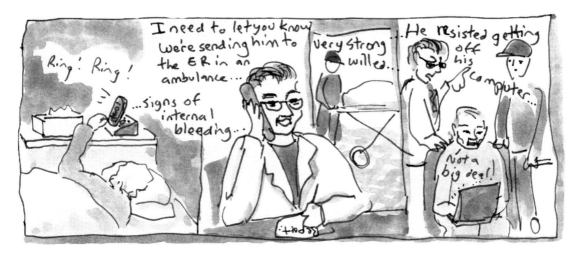

In the ER they discovered that his blood glucose level was very low again: low enough to impair his ability to make sense of the world around him and be mentally coherent. When Steve, who was diabetic, went this low he felt spacy and light headed and needed to quickly drink juice to bring his blood sugar back up to normal. So the problem of getting Aubrey to stop writing and shut off his computer wasn't just a resistant attitude, it was a legitimate medical emergency (with a simple short term fix). I called Anu to fill her in. She got on the road as quickly as she could and met me in the waiting room outside the ER. We both theorized that the low blood glucose issue had probably been happening for a while. We had both experienced varying degrees of Aubrey slipping in and out of making sense or being very spacy and not following some basic conversational threads. We shared this observation with the people attending him at the ER. We all agreed that low glucose levels could now be a significant factor contributing to his inability to be cognitively alert, comprehend conversations, and understand what he needed.

The process of trying to find veins for an IV went on for over thirty minutes with no success. His forearms were very swollen with extra fluid, while his upper arms were emaciated, just skin and bone, requiring the use of a small child's blood pressure cuff.

Aubrey was clearly annoyed about being in the hospital, with all the drama of medical attention, and claimed that every morning his blood pressure was that low but through the day it would rise, so he felt there was nothing to worry about. He made efforts to explain his spiritual healing project again. He told Anu, me, and the ER nurse that he was getting very tired of having to deal with solid food and eating. Even nutritional smoothie mix drinks were "weighing him down." He said all this attention on the "animal body" disrupted his focus on what was most essential: the meditative process of "shifting consciousness to the light body." Writing, meditation, and saying his prayerful mantras of healing was his main way to access that higher state.

The nurses and doctors explained that because he was Code 1, they had to intervene.

Angela, summoned to join the party, found inspiration while riding down in the elevator.

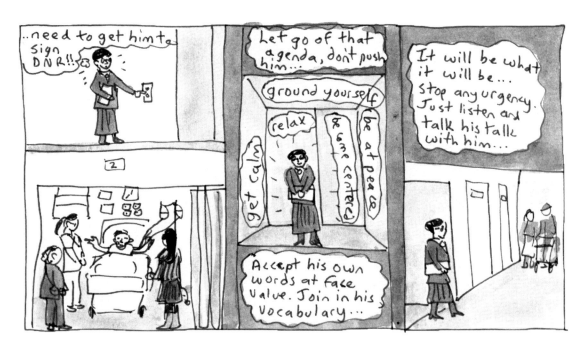

At his bedside, she joined Aubrey in using his vocabulary, listening and then repeating and reflecting back what he was explaining about his spiritual beliefs, healing with light, and true healing being in the mind. Anu and I witnessed their conversation, and a nurse did as well. Miraculously, Aubrey finally seemed to become clear that he had the choice to ask to not be given any further interventions, and that the mechanism for this was being taken off Code 1 status. He signed the DNR and the POLST (Physician Orders for Life-Sustaining Treatment), indicating that he was opting out of unwanted treatment such as being put on a ventilator or a feeding tube. He was clearly emotionally relieved and grateful, and we all breathed a sigh of relief.

Soon after that, he was deemed stable enough to be discharged. He gave the victory cry with his raised fist when told that all the tubes could be taken out of his arm and he could go home to Serenity Shores. I imagined that he would be so tired that he would sleep for the rest of the day, but the next time I got a phone call from the nursing home, it was a wonderful surprise!

Crossing the Finish Line

In general, lately, I've felt pretty dismal and grim, but it would be dishonest to overlook the miracles. Yesterday was a wild ride. The nursing home called in the morning to say Aubrey was being loaded (reluctantly) into the ambulance. After being stabilized in the ER, like last time, and finally choosing to stop engaging in all this "Code 1" intervention drama, he was allowed to go back to the nursing home. All he wanted to do, he said, was work on his book. I figured the day's adventure had worn him out, but he called me that evening at 7:30 pm to announce: "The book is finished! From front to back."

This morning I brought his first book to the nursing home so that he could reference the printed page while typing some minor edits he'd been wishing to clarify. In the hall I crossed paths with the residential care director who had called me the morning before. When I showed her *The Bluesiana Snake Festival* her jaw dropped. "So, he really IS a writer? A published author? He really knows what he's doing?" Yup, for real. Not just an old guy tapping away at his keyboard for the fun of it—not that that would not be enough to count. I swear it's what's kept him going this long. He says that healing is in the mind and that the creative process of writing is healing. To the soul, for sure. I'm not so sure about an imminent healing on the physical plane, but you just never know.

This afternoon, as I was leaving his room for the second time, after a visit including our son and my daughter, I mentioned that it was her dad's 60th birthday. That's when Aubrey, my second ex, got on the phone and called my daughter's dad, my first ex. I left the room and walked down the hall to the lilting tune of Aubrey singing "Happy Birthday" to him.

Another splendid connection this week was getting in contact with Aubrey's first wife, down in New Orleans. He hadn't wanted to bother her with any dour talk of cancer or death. He'd persisted in acting casual, as though there would be plenty of time left, not ruling out a resurrection that would allow for future visits, perhaps during Jazz Festival, perhaps a meal at the Napoleon House. But I felt it was time to reach out and find her. Our college's alumni office connected us. She called me. We talked on the phone for a long time. I dialed her up again, on my phone, in his room. They talked for a long time.

When he handed the phone back to me he said, very moved, "She said, 'Good-bye, honey, I love you.'" He said he never realized how much love there was, or how much love there was for him, until lately.

These are the precious moments that become available when people let down their guards and get real. In spite of all the facts I could list to justify feeling dismal and grim, I have to admit that life can also seem pretty sweet.

Author Interview

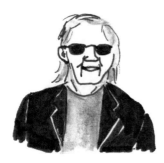

The Bluesiana Snake Festival, by Aubrey Bart
(2010, Counterpoint Press)

Herecome Hidden Dave Crossway—Jungian streetsweep working to support a writing habit (his novel *Lovers and Other Dirty Fighters* soon to be published soon as he got a publisher). Blowed from far look: shades, scarf, whichway hair. Comes off with the shades to hang out with Shushubaby

. . . Probably many a road scholar would testify this place makes good leavin and better comin back to . . . Place puts a hold on your soul, man, these streets call you like an old song . . . Yeah . . . Way downriver, heart of a swamp, she's a city made of music, down soft ground between memory and dream . . . Ain' no gettin down like the gettin down got down here, you gotta get it . . . Downriverway down womb of the land down subsealevel gets down as down gets, man—moon over this place puts heads thru changes . . . World comes in feedback rarefied down subsealevel, you get into this kinduva dream-am-I-dreamin-or-dream-dreamin-me sorta shuffle . . . Awta be official state headspace is what it awta . . . Deepspace propers down sameway pelicans get to be state bird, man, some quantum hype we're onto here . . . Lord knows people up and down these streets make living proof does being here contact buzz immaculate . . . Only makes sense people holdin offthewall karma would funk off here . . . Yeah, we've seen the saga . . . Pilgrim don't know you're a pilgrim, y'know, you're passin thru town . . . So you're passin thru and you're passin thru and you keep on passin thru, y'know . . . Days come round, you've gotten all but gone—somebody's pilgrim done gone new wave native . . . Happens here like it happens noplace else . . . Regular function at the junction all these people having moments people have only here . . . Popular creed comes off any excuse for a party or parade . . . That's howcome you see all this roleplaying, all these masquerade scenes around here . . . People get into it . . Unlived lives break loose on these streets, man, whatcha don't see here ain't happenin . . . Shadows outta closets put stories on the streets that's a preholy city true to form—man, you wear that out you ain't never lied . . . . . . Weird . . . . . . Coulda swore I caught that thought on the fly, now I'm flashin on some other time I dreamed it . . .

—Hidden Dave Crossway
Jungian streetsweep

Tell us about your career: "I've always done odd jobs to support a writing habit."

Tell us about your education: "I got a degree in history. Totally useless in the job market. My real education was on the road. I'm a Road Scholar."

Share a quote from your book: "Footfalls on the earthwalk make headway in all worlds."

What makes you most happy? "Bein' a dad."

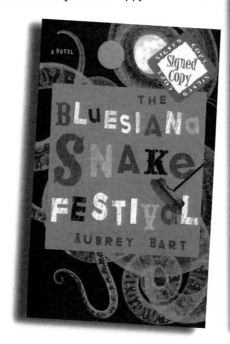

Odd Jobs that Supported a Writing Habit

New Orleans Taxi Driver

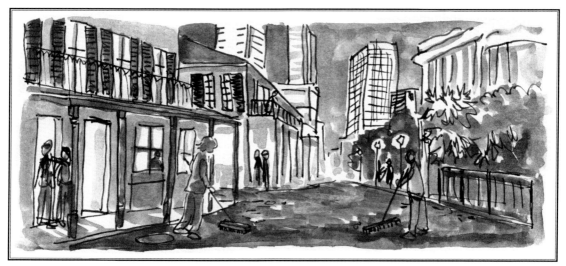

Street Sweep in the French Quarter

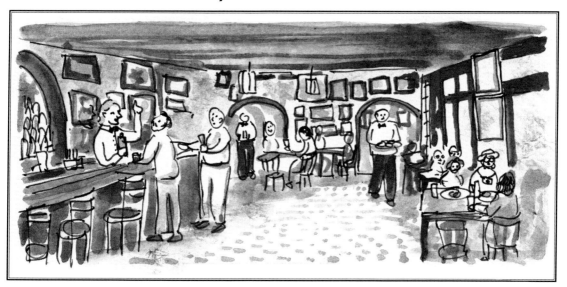

Bar Tender at the Napoleon House

Aubrey (the bar tender): "How do you like this music? Nice Beethoven, huh?"
Annoying customer (who was bragging about his musical prowess): "Yeah, man, I love it!"
Aubrey: "Well, actually this isn't Beethoven. It's Mozart."

6.

A Few More Dramas

Dad Goes Missing

Thursday afternoon, March 30th, I was in the waiting room of a new counseling office, sipping a complimentary cup of tea and trying to read a magazine, while Earl was in the next room, having his first meeting with a Licensed Clinical Social Worker (LCSW) to talk about his dad. Nurse Bea had come around noon to give Aubrey Reiki. He was dozing off by the time she left, when I had peeked in the door. He hadn't shaved for days and his palms looked unusually yellow. She sensed his time was close by his complete lack of appetite and grooming, how gaunt and tired he looked, the way he was breathing, and the way his eyes, half open, rolled back into his head when he dozed off. Even though he still wasn't interested to discuss death, she felt moved to say some things she wanted to say, for closure, for her own sake. She thanked him for their friendship and wished him peace and tranquility.

In some ways, even though they were close in age, she thought of him as a son, and she was a confidant he trusted. When things were rocky in our unstable relationship, she was the person in whom he confided, but she always treated both of us with respect and compassion, so I never felt judged. Now, at the end, she was a great person to have on our team. Getting Earl in to talk with a counselor was putting one more support structure into place; hopefully this first appointment would establish a useful relationship that would help him in the days to come.

My cell phone rang, interrupting this peaceful reflection. It was Anu, and she was very upset! Rhia had just called from the hospital. Things were happening that surprised us all. Aubrey was not where any of us expected him to be, and there was a lot of confusion and anger about what had just taken place. Apparently, some dots had not been connected between Aubrey, Serenity Shores, Small Brick Hospital, and the oncologist's office. Anu described Rhia's search.

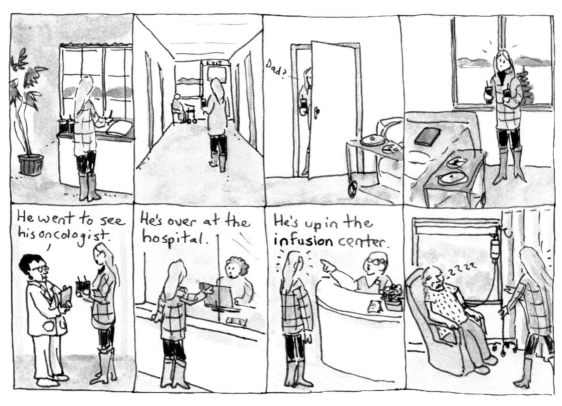

He went to see his oncologist.

He's over at the hospital.

He's up in the infusion center.

"Dad! *What are you doing here? What were you thinking?*" Rhia asked, when she found him.

He explained that he was getting an IV of Prednisone (or at least he remembered the doctor saying that word), and maybe a blood transfusion. But really it was an immunotherapy infusion. None of us in the family realized that Aubrey still had that oncology appointment on the calendar, nor that it would lead to more treatment. When he'd asked for no more medical interventions or treatments as of Monday, we'd assumed that was a "stop work" order for all further treatments. When questioned, the Infusion Center nurses said that he had agreed, had been perfectly clear minded, and that it was his choice. In fact, according to one, he still had "a chance of recovery."

I lost my temper over that one. For the first time ever I expressed anger, out loud, in person, in a formal institutional setting. (Of course it didn't help.) Earl, who had come along, later admonished me that people will listen more and respect your point of view more if you don't speak from a position of anger and accusation. He also chastised me for not letting him speak up, and said he would have been more level headed and effective. (I'm sure he was right.)

The next day, when Anu, Rhia, and I gathered in Aubrey's room, he said he was very proud of Earl for wanting to speak up for him. Then he explained what happened, from his point of view: when told that he had an appointment, he got into the van without protest, having learned that it wasn't going to do any good to resist being transported. He thought his choices on Monday had simply been nullified by the mysterious and powerful "medical system." He said he tried to explain the kind of inner spiritual healing work he was doing, but his oncologist didn't seem to understand. They "talked in circles for a while," the oncologist talking about immunotherapy, Aubrey about spiritual healing. The oncologist conceded that he didn't understand what Aubrey was talking about, but what he *could* offer was immunotherapy, and that there was "a good chance it would help."

"The doctor said I was *overdue* for a treatment. He said I was *behind schedule*," Aubrey explained. Even though other doctors had given him advice to stop or delay treatment, he felt anxious and worried that he had made a bad choice that had set himself back. Without the support of Anu or Rhia or me to be translators and advocates, he felt that he was being urged to get back on track and get immunotherapy in order to give himself the best chance of improving his health. He said he felt tired of talking in circles and finally went along with what he thought his doctor thought he should choose.

We asked him if he was aware that continuing immunotherapy was a completely different plan than we thought he wanted on Monday. It involved putting more chemicals into his body. He said he didn't really want any more chemicals. We asked him if he was aware that he was going to have side effects.

"Well, the doctor told me those are all treatable," he explained. But to him, "treatable" meant "fixable," in other words, he could be made to "feel better" again. We explained that "treatable" implies that the medical people have more procedures they can do, such as giving him more medicines, more hospitalization, more blood draws, more tubes in his arm, but with no guarantee of improvement, and did he want that?

He said no, he was tired of all of that, and frustrated by it. He said he felt utterly exhausted. He said that he thought he was finished with all of that as of his POLST and DNR paperwork on Monday. Then he waved a new piece of paper at us, which listed several new appointments for blood draws. "It shows here that now I have to go in *every week* for another blood draw!" He exclaimed, visibly upset. He thought that he was mysteriously back on some kind of conveyor belt where he had to show up and do what he was told by those in authority.

Oh, how I wished that Hospice had been engaged already!

Gallows Humor
(to the rescue)

Friday, March 31st, family met in the living room. I'd arranged the meeting because of feeling alone in trying to figure out some decisions. I wanted everyone to start talking and weigh in with their opinions.

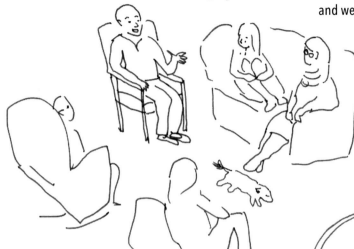

A volunteer from the cancer resource center facilitated the conversation.

The little dog walked around and around and then lay down exactly in the middle between all of us, and slept.

The volunteer explained about the process of cremation and asked where or if we wanted to spread the ashes.

We had not discussed this before.

We explained that the beloved had told us we could flush them down the toilet, but we didn't think we'd do that.

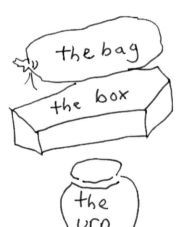

the bag

the box

the urn

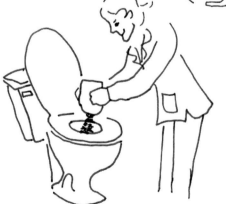

contains human bits

cremaines

heavy

The volunteer said the ashes would come by registered mail.

The box would be heavy.

Someone would have to sign for it.

176

Earl and Rhia, contemplating this scene, supplied narration:

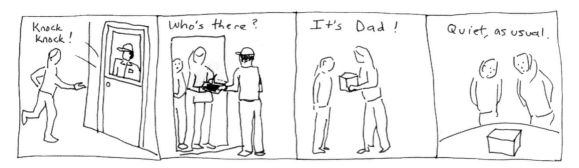

Suddenly we were all laughing so hard we were crying!

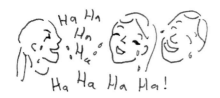

Dress Rehearsal of Death

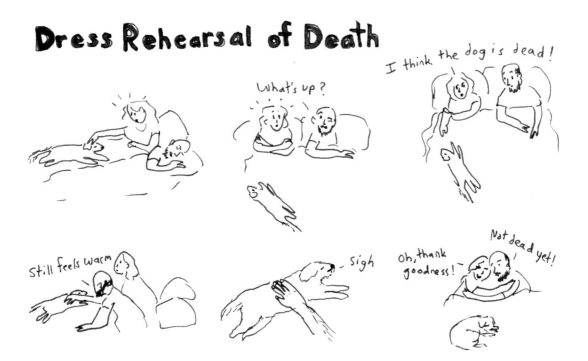

Hospice Begins

Friday, March 31st, Rhia carefully explained to her dad, in simple words, that it actually was *his choice*, that no one could *make* him do more treatments, and if he didn't want them he could "Just Say No!"

Aubrey straightened up from his hunched over position and very enthusiastically said "Yes! Make it stop! Can you tell that to everyone? Can you make sure The Matron knows?" He asked us three times to tell her this. We reassured him we would tell everyone who needed to know that he did not want any more treatments!

Rhia then described Hospice in very simple words: what Hospice could do to help him feel comfortable, and that with Hospice he could live right here in his own room and not have to go back to the hospital anymore. Aubrey said that sounded good. Anu and I spoke with The Matron and asked her to notify Hospice, but Serenity Shores could not get in touch with his primary care doctor before the end of the business day, so starting Hospice had to wait until Monday. (At least he still claimed to have no pain!)

Rhia visited him again late that afternoon, and texted me a warning: if I should happen to visit him with Earl, please be aware that Aubrey's face looked strikingly jaundiced.

Over the weekend he didn't feel like eating anything, the internal bleeding was back, and he said he regretted the infusion. Anu and I spent the better part of the weekend drafting angry letters to Mrs. Diplomacy. She offered to meet us in person at Serenity Shores as soon as we could find a time that worked for Aubrey's primary care doctor to join us. She asked me to call Dr. Kay's nurse to figure out a meeting time. The doctor would be making the rounds on Tuesday, so it would be that morning. The purpose of the meeting would be to make sure everyone was on the same page with all the decisions.

Monday, April 3rd, Hospice began. There was a meeting in Aubrey's room with The Matron, a Hospice social worker, a Hospice nurse, Anu, and me. There were a lot of personalities to relate to and lists of questions for Aubrey to answer. I could tell by the look in his eye that he was on the verge of being overwhelmed. When asked if he had a religious affiliation he said "I'm non-denominational," which led to a discussion of his spiritual beliefs and what he was trying to do to heal himself. When asked if he had pain, he said no. When asked about his appetite he claimed to be eating well, yet he turned down the hot lunch that was brought in by a nurse.

Out in the hallway, for privacy, I shared my concerns with the Hospice people about his incongruous answer. They reassured me that they were trained to look as well as listen, and they'd seen him skip the meal. Their task was to try to honor what the patient wanted, but also to look out for him. They could tell, from much experience, what was going on. By sending a Hospice nurse to visit him daily there would be a continual assessment of his changes, his pain level, and ways to support him in this time of transition. I found that very reassuring.

Aubrey said he didn't want a Hospice nurse to start coming every day, that was too much visiting time. He said once a week would be sufficient. They made eye contact with Anu and me, and calmly explained that, at least in the beginning, a nurse would visit three days in a row to establish the connection.

On Tuesday, April 4th, Anu and I got to Serenity Shores before Dr. Kay started her morning rounds. Mrs. Diplomacy met us in the lobby and The Matron led us to a private meeting room. Dr. Kay soon joined us. Anu and I discussed our anger and dismay about the events of Thursday. We were offered reassurance that our complaints were not off-base and would be passed along to all who needed to know, and there would be a review of some kind at the hospital, and all of our feedback would help improve the system.

Meanwhile, down the hallway, in Aubrey's quarters, there was a new and different Hospice nurse than the one he'd met the previous day, who was asking him all the same questions. He felt confused by all the different visits and complained to me that Hospice seemed invasive after all. He didn't understand their start-up protocol, so I explained to him that things would soon settle into a predictable routine with the same nurse and that everyone really did have his best interests in mind.

The Hospice social worker was available for home visits, and I took her up on this offer, for my own sake, making an appointment for her to visit with Earl and me in a couple of days. I had wished for that support for all of us, all along, and I felt as if I could breathe easier knowing there were finally some "end-of-life experts" on our team. It would be a relief to be able to talk to someone in person, to ask anything I wanted, and to share my feelings openly with someone outside the family.

Honestly, I wasn't sure how I felt. I'd been so doggedly focused on dealing with the physical level of reality and taking care of the formal details that it was impossible to engage with or process any of it emotionally. When I observed Rhia in tears that day, I didn't feel anything except a mechanical social cue to offer a hug and words of comfort. I admitted how numb I felt and conceded that I wasn't the best person to offer anyone else much emotional support.

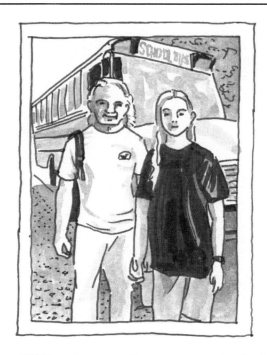

Update 4/4/17 I've been meaning to post an update for days, but the story line keeps changing, and it's been a challenge to summarize it while also dealing with the roller coaster ride.

The great news is, Aubrey finished his novel, on the evening of Monday, March 27th! I could hardly believe it, since he was just in the hospital that morning because of internal bleeding, low blood sugar, high heart rate, and super low pulse, same as the 15th-17th, when he was in the ICU at our local hospital.

He has decided he is ready to go off medications and stop immunotherapy treatment, and he asked for Hospice to be initiated. His body is fading fast, with evidence of liver failure, but his conviction in the power of conscious intention to heal on the level of heart/mind/spirit is strong. He explained that writing his book was a way to focus those healing intentions, and now that the book is finished, admits to being exhausted. He still claims to have no pain, which no one can comprehend. On Monday the ambulance driver said he could not believe that the critical vital stats matched up with the bright-eyed, calm, alert man he was transporting. Aubrey continues to inspire us, even as his body is fading.

Son's Last Visit

Wednesday, April 5th, was an unusual day for several reasons. For one, Steve was with us, having come to hear his daughter play in a concert Tuesday evening. After all of those meetings I had no energy left to go out with him, but he understood. Before driving home on Wednesday afternoon, he wanted to visit Aubrey, in case it might be their last visit. He knew there had been a lot of changes in the past few days and that Aubrey was languishing.

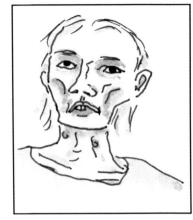

Earl hadn't been in for a visit since the day he and Ella shared photos and happy stories of his weekend away, and in some ways he wished that could be his last memory of his dad. But, while Steve was with us to bolster our spirits, I encouraged Earl to make one more visit, and he agreed. I prepared him by explaining about the retainer and a few other details: his dad wore a retainer with some false teeth that made his smile complete. It had somehow gone missing. (Aubrey was taking it out a lot; it no longer fit with the tumors in his mouth, anyway.) The point was, he looked a lot different without it. He was continuing to lose weight rapidly, and internal bleeding and possibly liver failure was causing jaundice, which made him look sort of suntanned. The room smelled strongly. He might be sleeping, or not interested to talk.

Earl set conditions that we would keep the visit brief, leave as soon as he asked, and that this would be his last visit. He said he would rather remember his dad as he used to look, not keep adding to his memory bank more images of the macabre decline. I agreed. We also decided that we'd go out for coffee and pastries at a bakery afterwards so as to add a bright spot to the day. Thus prepared, we set off.

When we got to Serenity Shores the Hospice nurse was finishing up, writing some notes. Aubrey was lying down, his eyes rolled back, his cheeks and temples shrunken in. We were going to quietly exit, when his eyes fluttered open enough to notice us, and we all greeted one another. After the opening dialogue, Steve said a few cheerful words, I asked Aubrey if he needed anything I could bring, and Earl said a few things. There were a lot of silences. After about fifteen minutes Earl signaled his discomfort, and, as we'd agreed, he got to decide how long the visit would last.

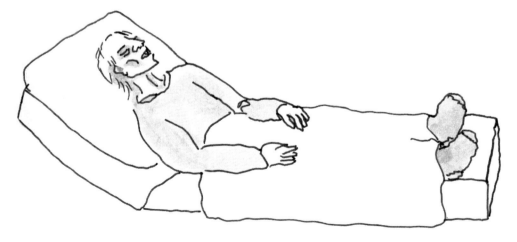

I explained to Aubrey that we were going to take Earl to the bakery for a treat, and he was glad to hear that. We all said our good-byes, then left him to rest.

When we were out at the bakery, a couple of friends and neighbors came over to say hi and ask how things were going. Warm cinnamon bun and soothing coffee in hand, my guard was down, and I answered truthfully about that momentous occasion, that it had been Earl's last visit with his dad.

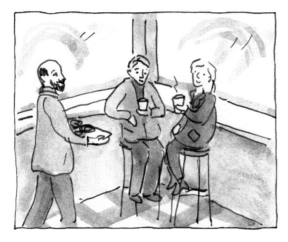

Being a small community, word spread. Later that evening I received a distressed and distressing message via Facebook. There was concern about Earl's decision to call that his "last" visit, and concern about my decision to go along with that. The message encouraged me to reconsider: shouldn't I take Earl to visit his dad as often as possible, in these last precious days, so as not to leave him prey to regret?

It's a fortunate coincidence that Glynda, the Hospice Social Worker, came to the house the next day. Some people have enough confidence to do what they feel is right without feeling anxious about what other people think, but I was not one of them, and I was both upset about the message and worried that I might have made a mistake, while at the same time feeling angry to be second-guessed by someone who really had no clue how raw and grotesque things had become. I didn't know how to respond.

Glynda was more than reassuring. She supported my decision, and said I should do what was right for my child; even if a child were much younger than thirteen she would encourage the parent to listen to what the child said and respect how they felt and trust that what they asked for was legitimate. It wasn't wrong or foolish for Earl to set that boundary. In the back of my mind I already "knew" what she was telling me, but the self-doubting part of my mind reveled in her coaching. The idea that I didn't owe anyone an explanation for how I was parenting was a perennial re-discovery, which I'd encountered in other situations. At least, quite often, I'd had Aubrey's opinion backing mine. Now I was in new territory; I'd never before parented a child whose other parent was dying.

Glynda also left us a booklet about changes in behavior and symptoms people may witness as their loved one's death approaches. I found Hospice's support very empowering, and I felt stronger and more confident going forward, knowing I didn't have to navigate this new and strange situation on my own. Glynda said a Hospice Bereavement Coordinator would be available to talk with Earl and me (and others in the family, if they chose) following Aubrey's death. They would be in contact with us right after the death and then monthly for the next thirteen months! Knowing this gave me so much comfort.

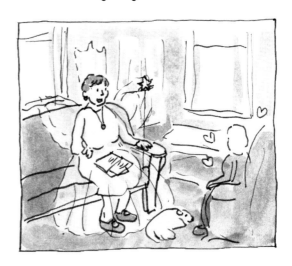

Facebook post Thursday, April 6

I've never done this before; I've never been so close to the epicenter of someone's dying process. So I'm learning as I go. The Hospice social worker's counsel was helpful today, helping me understand what I need to do and explaining what I am not obliged to do. But there are still the daily surprises, never knowing what the next text message or phone call will bring. And then it's up to me to decide how to respond, with as much grace and patience and poise as possible, while taking care of details I never took care of before.

The hardest part? Hard to say. I think today the hardest part was realizing how many people I am having to say no to. Because we've now engaged Hospice, suddenly everyone down the grape vine gets the message that the ship is going down, and everyone suddenly wants to visit and call and find out about what's been going on and connect over text, phone, and in person.

But since the beloved waited until the last minute to ask for Hospice, and has not yet been interested to discuss death and dying, the slow waning period is already over. We're already in the final days, folks, and it isn't pretty and nostalgic. The days for sentimental eye gazing and exchanging friendly reminiscences and imparting fatherly advice are over. We're done with the bringing of treats and eating being a pleasure. We're done with when taking a photograph together makes sense. It no longer makes sense because, trust me on this, this is not the way you want to remember him.

We're down to the way life looks when things are fragile, crusty, sallow, putrid, caving in, decimated, decomposing. Still among the living, but barely recognizable. Still having some good moments, but few and far between. The agitation, anxiety, and anger are kicking in. (Yes, I know there are ways to bring him relief, and I'm not in charge of choosing them.)

My main job lately is listening and receiving: directions on whom to call and who gets to visit, requests for payments and from people wanting to visit, taking calls from people who turn out to literally be characters from his first novel. It's kind of amazing. It's kind of like the movie *Big Fish*.

And I am sorry to tell you no, I can't call you from his room, I can't tell you yes please drive up and visit. I can't guarantee that if you do visit or call that he will be able to appreciate your efforts. I can listen a while, but I'm sorry, I don't know you like he knew you, and telling me instead of him must be a real letdown. I can only tell you he was so much more than he seems to be now, and thanks for all the best wishes and prayers. I'm glad to know how loved he is. Thank you, and good night.

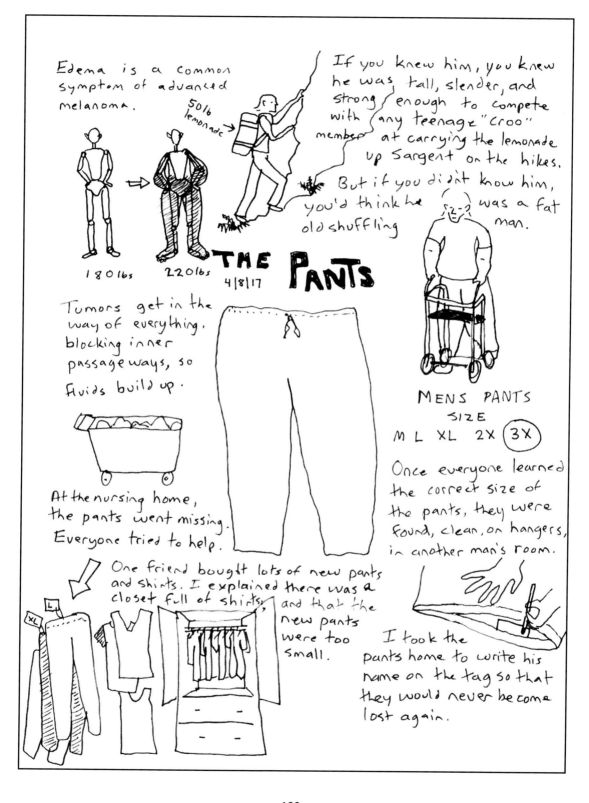

Edema is a common symptom of advanced melanoma.

If you knew him, you knew he was tall, slender, and strong enough to compete with any teenage "croo" member at carrying the lemonade up Sargent on the hikes.

50 lb lemonade

180 lbs   220 lbs

But if you didn't know him, you'd think he was a fat old shuffling man.

THE PANTS
4/8/17

Tumors get in the way of everything, blocking inner passageways, so fluids build up.

MENS PANTS SIZE

M L XL 2X (3X)

Once everyone learned the correct size of the pants, they were found, clean, on hangers, in another man's room.

At the nursing home, the pants went missing. Everyone tried to help.

One friend bought lots of new pants and shirts. I explained there was a closet full of shirts, and that the new pants were too small.

L
XL

I took the pants home to write his name on the tag so that they would never become lost again.

Pulling the Tumor

Wednesday, April 12th, at 3:30 in the morning, a nurse called from Serenity Shores to report that Aubrey had fallen, and because of all his extra water weight she and the other night nurse couldn't lift him. An ambulance was on its way. The attendants got him back into bed. I called Anu to let her know that, even though there wasn't anything we had to do. We were so glad he didn't get taken to the hospital. The nurse called me back to make sure we agreed with that.

Thursday, April 13th, at 6:00 a.m., the phone woke me up and again it was Serenity Shores. The Matron reported that Aubrey was hell-bent on pulling a massive tumor out of his mouth. He'd been pulling at it since midnight. The situation had turned from a fruitless endeavor into a medical emergency. He was bleeding so much that she couldn't just let him stay in his room and had to call an ambulance. Perhaps I might come over and help talk some sense into him?

I drove right over, and joined her and the chorus of nurses who were telling him not to do it.

There was blood everywhere: on bedding, towels, his clothing and hands. He sat on the edge of his bed with a focused look on his face, purposefully and relentlessly pulling at the unwanted thing which had been growing bigger and bigger inside his mouth.

We each took turns explaining that if he didn't stop he was going to rupture veins and might choke or bleed to death. Undeterred, he persisted. The ambulance and a Hospice nurse were on the way.

Alone with him for a few minutes, avoiding contact by using a garbage bag, I gingerly lifted the bloody towels from the floor and bed into the little garbage can from his bathroom. When I picked it up again to put it back in the bathroom it was as heavy as the gallon jugs of spring water I'd been bringing him.

The ambulance attendants arrived with the gurney and loaded him into the back of the vehicle. I promised The Matron I'd see if he could stay in the special Hospice room up at the hospital: for his sake, and to give her nurses a break!

She confided that in her whole career in elder care she'd never met someone as stubborn and strong willed as Aubrey! He certainly has that side to him, I conceded. Then we agreed it was debatable how much of his current behavior was conscious. He seemed to be out of his mind. He talked rationally, yet his actions were obviously not. He seemed to be beside himself, on autopilot. We shook our heads at what else we could have done to help him stop. Then I drove to the hospital.

Meanwhile, Carpenter Man came to visit Aubrey, as he'd been doing most mornings. He found out about the ambulance, so he showed up at the hospital soon after I got there. It was a huge relief to have a friend with me who was equally shocked by the novelty and audacity of the situation. Sitting in the waiting room together until we could enter the ER, we discussed Aubrey's amazing ability to not feel pain, or at least to not be fazed by it. Could doing yoga and meditation for decades give a person this ability to rise above it? At least one ER doctor conceded that this was a possibility.

In the ER they stopped the bleeding and asked him if he understood that he should not pull at the tumor any more. They were trying to deduce whether he had been conscious of his own efforts. He glanced over at me. He said he'd been told it was wrong and had been "caught being a bad boy."

Anger and disgust flowed through my body. I felt myself being cast, as I had been so many times in the past by this man, into the ridiculous role of "the adult who had tried to control him," who had told him what-not-to-do, and I was really done with that.

To handle being with him and witnessing what he had been doing drew upon every bit of training I'd had as a parent: dealing with exploding poopy diapers without flinching, learning to deal with wounds and bleeding and vomit without gagging, not turning away, because I was the adult-in-charge.

As soon as I could, I split to go take a shower and get Earl up for school. Needless to say I told him nothing about the incident except that his dad was alive and being taken care of, and no, Earl didn't need to go and visit him in the hospital. I just told him about the nice Hospice room we were trying to arrange.

Later in the day Carpenter Man called me and described holding Aubrey's bloody hand through the surgery; the doctor had basically stitched the thing back into place. Other than a local shot of anesthetic, as a dentist might give, Aubrey had refused further painkillers.

There was some debate about whether or not Serenity Shores could or should take him back, and in the end his choice to avoid all forms of treatment settled the matter: insurance wouldn't pay for the Hospice room at the hospital unless he were receiving some form of treatment, such as morphine. Fortunately (for us and him) when the hospital called the nursing home to see if they would take him back, The Matron agreed. So, back to his room he went.

I felt badly for the nurses there, and ever so slightly guilty for having failed to work it out for them to not have to deal with him again.

In the past, I'd enjoyed some high spiritual moments of togetherness with this man, but now I just felt disgusted, tense, and distant, derailed from all positive emotional connection with him.

Fortunately, Anu and Rhia were in a different headspace. They teamed up with one another to hold vigil by his bedside, together and taking turns, along with several of his friends.

Late that afternoon, the Hospice nurse called me at home and said there were signs that Aubrey might pass away within the next two hours. So I went back to Serenity Shores.

When I got there, he was sitting up and talking with Anu about transcending the cancer and healing his body. I left them to it, having neither the patience to listen nor the generosity of spirit to be cheerful. I didn't feel like going along with pretending that his death wasn't imminent. His words didn't seem profound, to me; they seemed to be about trying to maintain mental control and avoid surrenderring to the present reality.

So I went back down the hall to talk with The Matron about more business. We all knew Aubrey wanted to stay in his private room, but she explained that with the weekend approaching, when staffing would be lower, he would need to be moved to the west wing so as to have more supervision and care. That made sense, I agreed. Besides, it would probably be a good thing to have a new crew of nurses, and be a relief for those on the east wing who had witnessed that morning's drama.

Meanwhile, Mark and Betty and their daughter and her husband were all on the road, driving as fast as they could, desperately hoping for one last visit.

Different Perspectives

Friday, April 14th, Aubrey's relatives arrived. I'd warned them the journey was unlikely to be worth their efforts, and besides, I had no energy left for playing hostess. Thank goodness Anu and Rhia did, so they all had some quality time connecting with one another and visiting Aubrey's new room at Serenity Shores. Miraculously, they reported that he rallied for a heart-to-heart conversation with each of them. The Hospice nurse explained that near the end it was not unusual for even a very ill patient to have an energy surge, to suddenly become eager to eat, or alert and able to talk and connect meaningfully with loved ones. Uncle Mark told Earl a few more funny stories, including one about Aubrey stealing their mom's car one night, banging it up, but getting it repaired by morning so she never found out!

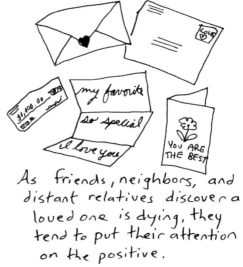

As friends, neighbors, and distant relatives discover a loved one is dying, they tend to put their attention on the positive.

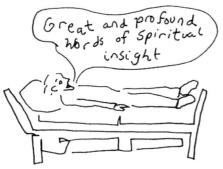

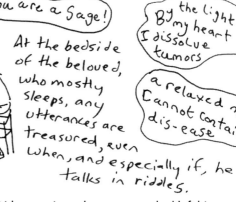

Anu wrote down some of the comments Aubrey made which seemed significant: he spoke of Jesus and the resurrection, of planning a trip to New Orleans, and of dreaming that an old college friend stood at the foot of his bed inviting him to come travel. He still didn't talk about dying, but it was easy to attribute symbolic meaning to his words.

I was still in a funk of resentment and disconnection, but trying to keep it to myself, using cartooning to privately work out my feelings on paper. Having so recently witnessed those gruesome scenes and put up with his stubbornness, I didn't feel the fondness and admiration other people were expressing. I felt angry with him for past situations as well, yet sad and ashamed to not behold him in the light of love.

Friday evening, when everyone had left his room except for Rhia, I went in to see how things were going. The west wing was abuzz with activity, patients in beds and wandering the hallway, hard-working nurses unable to keep up with all the calls for help. Aubrey's new room was larger than the previous one. The view was nothing special, but Anu had placed a pot of yellow tulips on the windowsill. The bed was accessible from both sides, which was handy. A nurse was trying to help him get comfortable by tugging at the sheet under him to try to move his heavy body into a different position. His utter helplessness and obvious discomfort prompted me to put aside my small-mindedness and do what I could to help.

Sainthood

The closer he came to death, the more he was swooned over; women from distant states, countries, and continents sang his praise. I still had a few incidents to forgive.

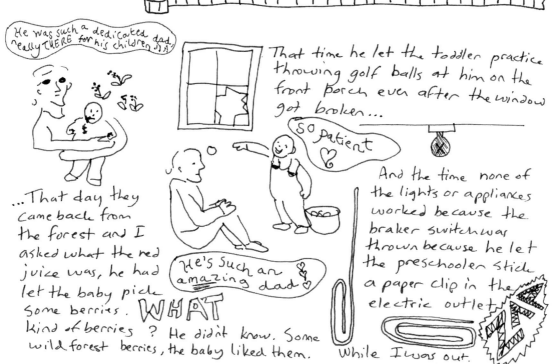

He was such a dedicated dad, really THERE for his children !!!

...That day they came back from the forest and I asked what the red juice was, he had let the baby pick some berries. WHAT kind of berries? He didn't know. Some wild forest berries, the baby liked them.

He's such an amazing dad ♥

That time he let the toddler practice throwing golf balls at him on the front porch even after the window got broken...

SO patient ♡

And the time none of the lights or appliances worked because the braker switch was thrown because he let the preschooler stick a paper clip in the electric outlet. While I was out.

Tugging at the sheet from the other side, I joined in to no avail. The nurse had to go, so Rhia and I took over in trying to follow his directions about where to place pillows. He denied he felt pain, but he was obviously uncomfortable. I tried doing Reiki but he remained agitated. Rhia and I talked privately. Then, avoiding the word "pain," we carefully explained that trying just a tiny bit of morphine might help him: because if he was not so preoccupied on trying to find the right position for his body, then he could put more attention into his prayers and meditations. At last he consented. We were silently victorious, exchanging glances of relief, and went to find a nurse right away before he could change his mind.

It took a while before the shot could be administered (more paperwork and looking up things on the computer), but at last they came in with the syringe. Thankfully, the drug helped him relax. Then I went home for the night. Aubrey asked Rhia to stay. She asked him if he felt fear of dying and he didn't say. She rested on the other bed. Every time a nurse came to check on him, he'd ask if his daughter was okay, keeping his focus on his concern for her.

By morning the Hospice nurse's prognosis changed to, "He'll probably make it through the weekend." It's a good thing others could attend to him, because my attention would be needed elsewhere.

Grand Pops Does It Again!

Facebook post Saturday, April 15

Aubrey is still with us! Hospice thought he was close two days ago, but he continues to surpass expectations. Thankfully his brother and sister-in-law and their daughter made it in time to have one more visit, and he miraculously rallied enough to join in conversation.

At his most recent ER visit, though talking very slowly, Aubrey lectured from the gurney to a captive audience of ER doctor, hospice nurse, two social workers, and his daughter's mom and me, about the misdeeds of the medical-industrial complex making profits off cancer treatments, and the value of the nine part video series, "The Truth About Cancer." Back at the nursing home he was moved to a different wing where there is more intensive nursing support.

Meanwhile, today, my dad, in ring two, pulled off surviving a 4th heart attack, and will most likely go home after a night in the local hospital. All of this almost-but-not-quite behavior does make way for candid conversations. Glad my folks celebrated their 52nd anniversary together yesterday.

And finally, in ring three, my children and Steve and I decorated eggs, met our new summer housemate-to-be, and attended a little circus at the college this evening.

Thank you all for the best wishes and prayers.

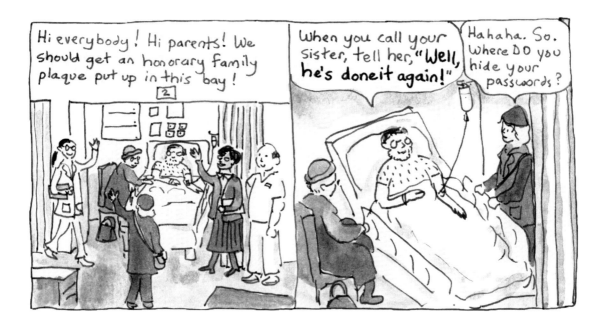

Easter Sunday

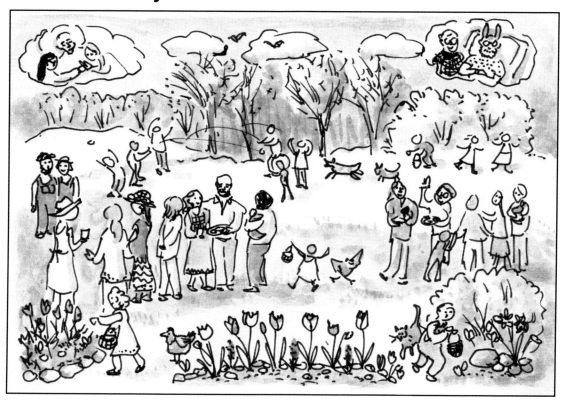

Sunday, April 16th had three situations going on at once, each of which could have commanded the mood of the whole day. My dad was still in the ICU, my mother by his side, nothing to be done but wait and stay under observation. I brought them a little Easter basket, and he kept the bunny ears headband on even when the nurses came in. Meanwhile, Aubrey was in his new room with Anu, Rhia, and Nurse Bea beside him. Even his old nurses from the east wing came to sit with him during their breaks. So, with all patients accounted for and attended by other people, I spent Sunday afternoon with Steve and Earl at the annual community potluck at a friend's house. As well as yummy food and the chance to catch up with a bunch of our friends, there was an egg toss, an egg hunt, and lots of happy children, dogs, cats, and chickens running around. Spring flowers were in bloom and the air was sweet and mild.

After the party, Steve and I walked Tucker dog over to Small Brick Hospital. We took turns waiting outside with him in the picnic area while the other one went inside to visit my parents. My dad needed to stay for the night, but he enjoyed some coffee cake and admired the dyed eggs.

Early in the evening, Steve left for home. When my mom walked over from the hospital after dinner, I drove her home for the night.

Finally, Earl and I got into "cozy time" mode. We put on our pajamas and started watching a documentary about whales. We agreed it had been a nicer day than many in recent memory. Nevertheless, all the comings and goings and relentless intensities had left my mind rather frazzled, so I took some sleeping medicine just to be sure to get a deep night's rest.

A Portal Opens

After sudden and monumental events, people often remember in detail the place they were when they found out the news. Earl and I were at home in our pajamas, watching a newborn whale taking its first exploratory swim alongside its mother, when the phone rang at 9:40 p.m. on Easter Sunday. Anu spoke in a soft voice: "He's gone."

She and Rhia were in his room. They'd been there all day, massaging his arms and legs, swabbing his lips with water, giving him flower essences, singing and chanting prayers. His eyes were open but he couldn't see. He said no words, slipping in and out of sleep. They were exhausted, had retreated to the adjacent bed where they rested, and were talking quietly with one another. At one point they looked over and noticed his chest was no longer rising and falling.

Stillness, silence, time on pause. There was a blessed hush about the atmosphere that neither wanted to spoil by calling a nurse. A sacred portal had opened. The beloved had departed. All worldly troubles seemed less real, just stories. Neither Earl nor I felt bereft upon hearing the news. He said he felt some sadness, but mostly relief. I felt relief more than anything. Aubrey's soul had finally taken flight from that very broken body. There was a sense of wonder and awe, knowing that someone we knew so long and well had passed "beyond the veil."

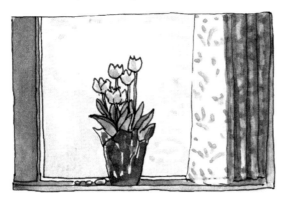

Earl and I talked. We imagined his dad in some other dimension, welcomed by angels, beings of light, maybe some sort of spirit guides. We imagined him somewhat confused and startled by being bodiless but still conscious. We imagined them reassuring him that they were holding the space for him, supporting him in the transition just as midwives and doulas support a mother and baby during birth. But beyond the realm of imagination and mental conjecture, it was a total mystery. Where was he now? Still a separate being, or "one with all of consciousness," a water drop absorbed into the ocean? We talked until we both felt ready to write in our journals and sleep.

Rhia and Anu lay on the other bed in Aubrey's room, suspended in the stillness and silence, until the nurse on-duty made the rounds and discovered what had happened. Then the clock started ticking again, galloping into the meeting of deadlines and the activation of protocols at full tilt.

When a patient dies, there is only a short window of time a nursing home can keep a dead body on the premises. Normally, a family has a contract with a funeral home, and one phone call trips the switch and the funeral home takes over from there. But this was not our plan. Our friend, The Farmer, had offered to help for free, "bypassing the for-profit Death Industry," so we would only have the cost of the cremation. He had experience. I'd gone to the Town Office with him and obtained the necessary papers, and he had obtained the body bag and the requisite box from the crematorium. Hospice would be called to witness the death, then the body would need to be kept in cold-storage for forty-eight hours, then a doctor would need to sign the death papers. After that, cremation could take place.

That night, since I was already under the influence of the sleeping medicine, unable to drive, I stayed at home with Earl. The only thing I remember was being awakened briefly by a phone call from Hospice saying the nurse was on his way to Serenity Shores.

Exit Strategy

The next morning, I met Anu at Serenity Shores to collect Aubrey's belongings from the room. That's when I heard the story of what had happened during the night. She actually began by laughing! When she told me, I couldn't help but laugh as well. The nursing home called Hospice, and Anu called The Farmer, but he didn't get the message right away, so there was anxiety at Serenity Shores. Finally, in the wee hours of the morning, he arrived in a pick-up truck with the bag. He met Anu, the Hospice nurse, and others from the nursing home inside. He was expecting to find a gurney on the premises, and the nursing home expected him to have brought one. So they had to use a wheel chair.

A nurse from the other wing looked out the window in time to see the bag being loaded into the truck. Alarmed, she called The Matron. "There's a guy here with a pickup truck! Aubrey's leaving in a pickup, in a body bag!" The Matron, at home asleep until this call, was informed of and on board with our unconventional plan. Yet she couldn't help getting a little chuckle about the way it all came down.

"Perfect. As he should," she replied.

Anu and The Farmer had a long hug (with tears in their eyes, I imagine), then he got in the truck, and off it went, into the dead of night. This sounded like a scene right out of a story Aubrey might dream up and write! Anu and I agree that if he were looking on from above he would be most amused.

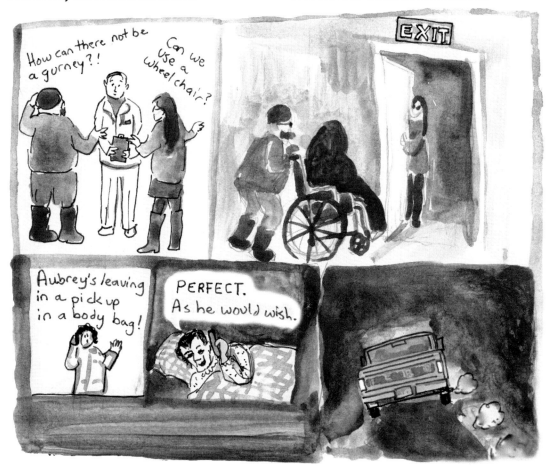

191

7.

Carrying On

What Happens Next?

One of the stupefying facts which one encounters after a loved one has died is that life just keeps on going. We, the living, are left to carry on. The earth somehow keeps turning. New events take place that are also considered important, such as births, graduations, concerts, sporting events, and classes at school, in spite of the fact that for you everything is still colored by death.

Death is as universal as birth, yet how we experience the death of a loved one and how their absence changes our lives is as individualized as it gets. What happens next is different for everyone; there are different feelings, different tasks, and different ways of dealing with all of that.

In our case, each of us had risen to the occasion and pulled together as a team, each with different roles to play to get through Aubrey's illness and dying. After his death, each of us withdrew back into our own corner, confiding in other people–or not confiding at all. There was barely any communication between the rest of us, so I can only speak for myself regarding what happened next.

During the first week, I found myself charting each day in relationship to the date of his death: Monday: Day 1 after Aubrey's Death; Tuesday: Day 2 After Death; Wednesday: Day 3 A.D., and so on.

Birds were singing spring songs, flowers were coming into bloom. My dad was still in the hospital, my mom still needed rides. The dog still needed to be walked and fed and given insulin shots every twelve hours. Earl went out to the back yard and dug a hole so deep the dog couldn't climb out of it whenever he fell in. Then he got a five day cold and slept through the week on the couch. I had a Monday morning appointment to get the snow tires off my car. Later in the week there was a snow storm. It was all very surreal.

In the beginning, I didn't feel sadness or loss, just fatigue and relief. Aubrey wasn't suffering anymore. The relentless medical emergencies were over. There were no more phone calls from the nursing home.

As time passed, different feelings arose: anger, sadness, resentment, cynicism, and nostalgia among them. A Hospice Bereavement Coordinator called the house right away, and soon after that we got a letter in the mail along with a booklet about grief, loss, and healing, describing some of the feelings and issues people may encounter soon after the death of a loved one. That phone call, letter, and booklet all reassured me that Earl's quiet withdrawn behavior and my own mixedup feelings were normal; everything we were going through was normal. Normal, normal, normal. That didn't mean it wasn't confusing, just that even the confusion was normal.

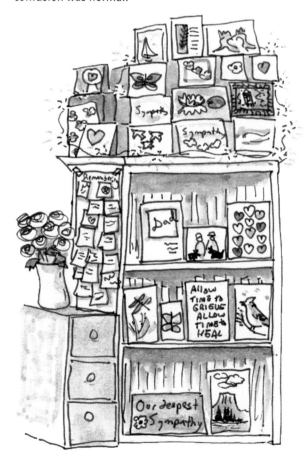

DIY Funeral Director

Each day of the first week following the death was exceptionally longer than normal, taken over with novel tasks. What might those be? I figured this out as I went along. In the modern world there are so many entanglements to undo when a person dies!

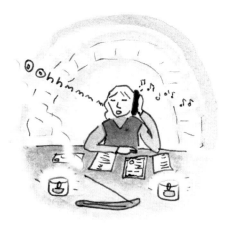

All the checklists I found online were incomplete and had tasks that didn't apply in Aubrey's case. (For example, there were no stocks or bonds, no life insurance policy, and no club memberships to cancel.) It was frustrating to figure out what needed to be done and by when. If my state, country, and modern society expected certain official, legal, and practical business matters to be dealt with postmortem, why wasn't there a definitive list to consult and check off?

When I mentioned my frustration about this on Facebook, someone didn't catch my drift and encouraged me to make the novel post-death period "magical," and to "make it my own." Although this comment was meant to be supportive, I felt cynical: as far as I could tell, there was no way to make these business-related tasks "magical." Perhaps I should have lit a candle and burned some incense while waiting on hold for an hour with the insurance company?

What I didn't realize, until days later, was that I was legally operating *as* the funeral director. I finally figured out that if we had paid to engage a funeral home, the funeral director would have taken care of–or at least coached me through–much of this, and in retrospect I might have preferred that guidance to the "Do It Yourself" version. Unless someone has the free time and energy to commit to a week or more to driving all over the place and dealing with all sorts of paperwork and making a lot of phone calls, they'd be better off working with the help of a funeral home and funeral director, if only for someone to lean on for advice.

Then again, we saved over $700 by not doing it in the conventional commercial manner.

Some tasks, such as getting the certified death certificate before the cremation, were time-sensitive. Another reason to do some tasks sooner than later was the unfortunate modern phenomenon of "identity theft." I learned that you should buy multiple copies of the death certificate and inform organizations such as banks and credit card companies about their client's death. (Even though I did that, Aubrey continues to receive monthly statements from Medicare and offers for lower interest rates on his canceled credit card!) Some of the nicest conversations I had in the first week were with strangers whom I called to settle these matters. The editor from the newspaper, the vitamin and mineral saleswoman, the operators at Social Security, the phone company, and AAA, all took time (even if it was because they were following company protocol) to offer their condolences.

Other tasks were not time-sensitive, so some family members might have helped, but their priority was on the emotional processing side of things, and they said they couldn't help *yet*. But I wanted my life back. I wanted all of the Aubrey-related "homework" to be done. The knowledge that it had to be done *eventually* felt like a tension I couldn't escape from until it *was* done. Since I was the one impatient to finish this homework, I chose to plug along instead of delegating and accepting the slower pace at which others might have completed these tasks.

(Another) Incomplete To-Do List

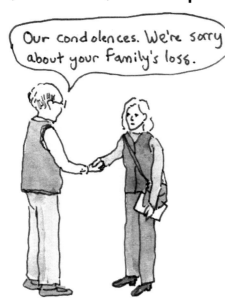

Our condolences. We're sorry about your family's loss.

Monday 4/17
- email and call Aubrey's closest friends and relatives
- post announcement on Facebook (*after* phone calls!)
- take death certificate paperwork to clinic
- leave it for primary care provider to sign
- edit and finalize obituary
- obituary and mug shot to newspaper, pay by the line
- notify Medicare, Social Security, state insurance

Tuesday 4/18
- get death certificate from the clinic to the Town Office
- go back to the clinic for one more signature
- drive Papa home from the hospital
- write generic thank you note and announcement of death
- email it to online fundraiser donors
- print copies of obituary and generic letter and thanks
- mail these to all who sent donations and cards by mail

Wednesday 4/19
- Sleep in? No! Town Office called: need to get certified copy of death certificate to crematorium ASAP
- get a fax of the notorized death certificate sent to the crematorium by 10 a.m. when the body arrives
- drive up to the crematorium before end of the business day to turn in certified copy of death certificate
- learn about, sign for, and collect cremains
- cancel Saturday's community supper at soup kitchen

Thursday 4/20
- banking: find out what to do with his account
- contact credit card company, cancel
- find lost post office box key
- turn in key, close box (keep forwarding mail)
- make plans to get car towed, donated for parts
- donate clothing to thrift store in other town

Friday 4/21
- court house: get paperwork regarding his will
- contact his cell phone company, terminate service
- contact car insurance and AAA, cancel
- contact AARP, cancel
- pay balance of room and board to nursing home
- contact vitamin and mineral supplement company, return unopened box for a refund

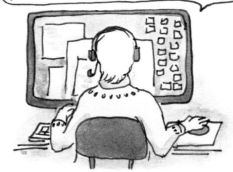

First, let me express our condolences for your loss. No, he didn't have any orders left to fill. My goodness, he certainly did purchase a lot in the past three months!

Love-Fest Lamentations

It was also a confusing time socially. My son's dad was dead. Did that make me a widow? There isn't a label for what to call a surviving ex-wife, nor any cultural expectation for her to grieve. And even when people did reach out in kindness, I sometimes felt cynical. I'd already "felt his loss" on the home front acutely in years gone by, but that grief wasn't public. By the time he died, Earl and I had already found our sea-legs in terms of being a fatherless household, so that wasn't a new challenge for us to encounter. After his death I didn't feel nearly the grief or loss that I'd endured during our twelve years of trying to be in a relationship. Still, his absence did leave a hole.

I had reserved the soup kitchen for a "celebration of life" potluck, but the others weren't ready to appear in public that soon, and I couldn't imagine doing it without them, so I canceled. Since none of us went to a church with any consistency, there wasn't an obvious built-in condolence community. I imagine many people we knew were just waiting to be told when and where to meet for a nondenominational memorial, but it was mid-summer before we offered them such an event to attend. By then the death was no longer headline news, and many who might have come earlier didn't have time to attend.

Nobody brought casseroles! I could have asked, but it seemed like asking for a kiss...if you've gotta ask, it isn't quite the same...and we'd been given so many handouts already...the donated meals, the soup kitchen fundraiser, the online fundraiser...many days later someone inquired if meal deliveries would be useful, but by then I was back to trying to eat according to a special diet, and asking others to be that careful just felt as if it would seem picky.

Mumsie, true to form, created baked goods: ingeniously rainbow-striped heart-shaped sugar cookies, a tin for Rhia and a tin for Earl.

During the first week, many people figured I must be overwhelmed by phone calls, so they, trying to be kind, didn't call, resulting in the strange phenomenon that only one person called. I could have called many people if I'd wanted a listening ear, but my feelings were too mixed up to talk about. I sent out a general email announcing Aubrey's death, and many people did email back. People to whom I'd mailed a paper thank-you letter and announcement, such as the mostly older generation who had chosen to send checks by mail instead of to donate electronically online, followed old-school etiquette by sending real paper condolence cards by mail. Earl and I appreciated them so much! I set up a little shrine on the bookcase in the corner of our living room.

In the modern world of social media, Facebook became the main medium by which most people shared their condolences. But, to my consternation, I was in such a funk that I couldn't receive their love: what surprised me the most as I read some messages was that I felt angry and disgusted! And it didn't feel like the kind of anger in the stages of grief over death and dying. (Besides, that list was meant to describe the experience of the dying person, it wasn't intended as a road map for the survivors.)

Why did people saying nice things about Aubrey trigger me to feel anger? Hadn't I been focusing on the positive in him and sharing that in all my posts to the world? Isn't it polite and natural to look for the positive in a person when mourning their death? What was wrong with me? Well, it seemed as if people were putting him up on a pedestal of perfection, expressing an almost cult-like level of awe. I'd been one of the closest people to him, and I knew there was more to the story. On the other hand, their feelings of love and admiration seemed honest, and I felt sad to not be joining in the love-fest. Perhaps what stung the most was that they still saw him as I used to see him, before we were married, back when I'd fallen in love.

How I Met Your Father

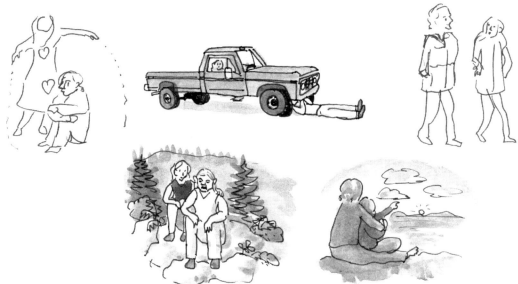

It was early spring.
The trees were just starting to bud.
The birds were beginning to sing.
Our romance didn't start off as a romance.
The affair began (as many do) as an innocent
friendship. We met in a Eurythmy movement class
at the Waldorf school where our daughters were in
Kindergarten. We (and everybody else) paired up
for an exercise: I walked around him, with my arms
outstretched, being "the encircling warmth of the
sun," while he sat on the floor in the role of "the pine
tree." During tea break we talked.

"Did you feel that?" he asked me, "It felt as if you
were seeing right into my heart!"
"I did feel that connection! Whatever happened, that
was amazing!"
"You bypassed my defense mechanism and came
right down through the chimney!"
"Some day I want to take classes to become an
energy healer."
"*Some* day? You're already *doing* it!"

It felt as if we were being drawn together to do some
important healing work.

We started going for walks so that I could confide in
him. A lifetime of secrets, hopes, and dreams found
a sensitive listening ear. He was kind, open-minded,
accepting of everything, and shocked by nothing. No
matter what I said he bore witness to my innocence.
He seemed to see right into my heart and soul–and
I into his. We'd both spent our lives being the one
in whom others confided. Now, in one another, we
discovered an equal peer. Perhaps if we'd left it at
that we could have remained close friends for life,
without all the hassles. (But it is impossible to erase
our past without erasing our son, so, no regrets.)

The old truck that took him away into the dead of
night reminded me of the first time he took me for
a drive. In order to start his old blue junker, he had
to lie down on the road, scootch under the front
between the wheels, and jerry-rig something. Right
away, gut instinct told me it wasn't a good idea to
pursue a relationship. Not that I was aiming for that
anyway. But things got complicated, as they often
seem to do between old souls who are here to work
out whatever karma they have left with one another.
He had sensitive eyes and a very nice voice.

I wanted the world to know that I honestly loved him; that it wasn't "just" an affair or a "transitional" relationship. So we got married right away, as soon as my first divorce went through. That's when the trouble began. Beneath the foot of rich top soil everyone else saw, there was a solid granite ledge. He never hurt me physically, but he would become lost in his old nightmares, suddenly seeming to forget who I was, no longer trusting me, questioning my motives with suspicion. It seemed as if I must be patient and gracious in all ways at all times, but still could be argued with and rebelled against at any moment. I felt as if I were his mother, not his wife, and he was a moody teenager who was sullen and withdrawn. Or perhaps he was two people: the one I had fallen in love with, and the passive-aggressive Evil Gemini Twin. I lived with perpetual anxiety and found no solace or comfort in the marriage. Our relationship was full of turbulence, with enough self-sacrifice, sabotage, and heartbreak to make a ridiculous movie. We got divorced soon after Earl was born. But we still loved each other, and the attraction didn't end. On our own, we each did a lot of "inner work" and made progress on acceptance and forgiveness.

The year Earl turned seven, it seemed as if starting over might be possible, as well as save us money by combining our resources. So we got married again! But when he moved in he said the house made him feel claustrophobic. He'd come and go as he pleased, leaving me with all the responsibilities. He made all his own meals and said I wasn't obligated to feed him. I felt as if I were running a boarding house and he was my bachelor tenant. To top it off, with his total annual income added to mine (even though he had debts for rent and his car and had just quit his bus job), Earl and I lost our health insurance. When I admitted what I was dealing with, and wondered if divorce was a cop-out, our family counselor said no, in fact, I would be doing myself–and him–a favor. "This is not how a healthy marriage or good parenting works. You're not wrong for expecting more." If anything, I'd been trying much too hard for much too long. Letting go of the marriage was a sane choice to make, and a relief. But, along with grief, I also felt more embarrassed than I'd ever felt before: with his mostly wonderful reputation, I, having initiated both divorces, looked quixotic. Hardly anyone could understand why I would let him go. Again!

Sorting through his clothing provoked many memories.

199

On the Way to the Crematorium

Wednesday, April 19th, at 10:00 a.m., three days after Aubrey died, was the reservation at the cremation. Anu and The Farmer drove up together, body bag in box, box in truck, while I completed the death certificate paperwork. (It turned out to take longer than anyone had anticipated, due to some procedural changes in electronic filing on the state level, but we got everything done just in the nick of time.)

I was still in a funk to the point of feeling almost toxic, so I didn't want to join them or impose my dour mood into their sacred space. Instead, I offered to drive up by the end of the work day to collect the box of cremains. It would be a long drive. A chance to reflect in private and maybe chill out a little. After all of the mundane tasks I'd done on Aubrey's behalf, there was some perverse pleasure in wrapping up this part of the chore list; a "once-in-a-lifetime" event, so to speak. Mentally, I did a brief scan of my surroundings to see if I "felt his presence," but I didn't. I was free to feel and think anything and it didn't matter; he was immune from it all. He was, in fact, immune from all manner of earthly problems. Another emotion emerged into my consciousness: envy. I envied him. Not that I knew at all where his soul was or what he was going through, but I imagined it to be a better place, like being on vacation. I felt stuck in the physical world.

Then something strange happened. When I plugged in my cell phone to charge it, music came out of the car's speakers. Because I was driving, I couldn't easily figure out which buttons to press to make it stop, and even at a stop light I couldn't make it stop! The music that was playing was titled "Songs of Innocence." But, I'd never downloaded that album onto my phone! The concept of innocence got me to thinking about a spiritual book that Aubrey and I had read. It had helped us learn about forgiveness, and "holy" relationships, and to feel more harmonious.

Now, I didn't want to strong-arm myself out of this current funk by denying the legitimacy of the feelings, but that funk, going on for days, was getting to be so constricting and heavy and uncomfortable to endure that I found at least a small willingness to see things differently. So I spoke some of the words I remembered from the book. "May I exchange these grievances for the miracles they obscure."

My other active choice that afternoon was to try an idea Anu had found and shared on Facebook that morning: while a cremation is taking place you offer up anything you'd like to have burned (metaphorically speaking) or transformed, and you also release the loved one with blessings and peace. I figured trying this couldn't hurt. I was the one hurting, after all. Maybe he was already at peace. Then I thought: what if he wasn't? What if he knew what was in my heart but had no way to fix it? How would it feel to know that someone was still angry with you but you had no more life left on earth with which to mend anything? Besides, do we have to be *perfect* to be remembered with love? Was I perfect? Certainly not! I remembered times that he had felt very sad and disappointed. Every uncomfortable memory and feeling that came up–blame, shame, anger, dismay, disgust, disappointment, and regret, to name a few–I imagined releasing into a purifying flame.

My grievances became much less interesting than the inspiring ideas that began streaming though my mind. By the time I reached the crematorium, the funk had dissolved like a bank of fog lifting, and even the actual landscape looked more beautiful. The crematorium was on the grounds of a cemetery (as they must be, by law) and the place was really lovely, with lots of trees, green grass, and spring bulbs in bloom. I parked and got out of the car. As I walked around looking for the director's office, I had a spring in my step and a smile on my face!

What to do while waiting at the Crematorium

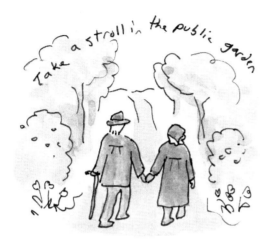

Take a stroll in the public garden

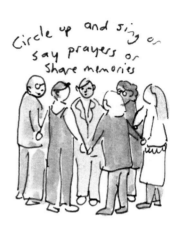

Circle up and sing or say prayers or share memories

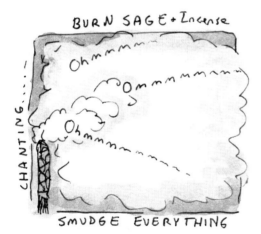

BURN SAGE + Incense

CHANTING.....

Ohmmmmmm

Ommmmmmm

Ohmmmmmm

SMUDGE EVERYTHING

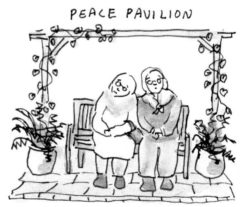

PEACE PAVILION

The director's office was near the furnaces, so I got to see inside the functioning inner sanctum of the place. He greeted me kindly, showed me around, then he handed me the box. As I was expecting, it was heavy! He explained that there was a little metal tag inside the plastic bag with the cremains and to be sure not to accidentally leave it if we spread the ashes in nature. There were other rules and regulations to follow as well, and yet more papers to sign.

Then I decided to tell him about the inspiration I got during the drive: to make a graphic memoir about everything: the cancer, the dying, even this! "For real?" he asked. "We'll see!" I replied. "Well, if you really do, I want to see it!" he said. "Certainly!" I promised, "Can I take a photo of these machines? For artistic purposes?" (He let me, but I decided to leave them out, after all.) We shook hands, then I drove home with the heavy box and a *much* lighter heart.

Grieving and Laughing

It wasn't a permanent attitude shift, but the healing had begun. When Sunday rolled around again (the one week anniversary), Earl and I were still living in an altered state–he with some symptoms of depression and anxiety, both of us very tired–but we were starting to take some baby steps to restore normalcy to our lives. While Steve attended his daughter's orchestra concert, we stayed home in our pajamas and finished that documentary about the baby whale taking its first swim. We reflected that we were emerging from the depths of the most difficult times.

The next weekend, Nurse Bea came over for tea. She talked about her special friendship with Aubrey, and about him confiding in her during our divorces. "He felt so responsible for what happened between you two. He shared all his regrets with me," she explained. I heard those words as if they were a message to me from Aubrey. It made me want to let go of any blame that was left in my mind and just send him love and best wishes. I hoped he was at peace.

The next day, Sunday–the two week anniversary of the death–Earl and I got dressed up and went along with Steve to hear his daughter's Senior Recital. It was such a pleasure to experience live music which was so well prepared and performed!

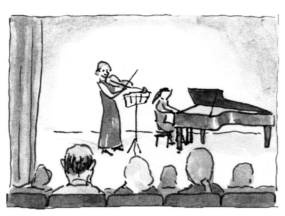

While it was true that we were emerging, it wouldn't be clear until I looked back months later just how much we were still under the influence of the dying time. Some days we felt "normal," but that was relative to the day before and it wasn't a steady incline. The next day, for no reason at all ("No reason except for *My Dad Died*," said Earl) we'd feel depressed and have a hard time getting out of bed. Small things could trigger us to feel angry, sad, or irritable. Looking back over the past half year, I can appreciate that one can't mentally fast-forward through grieving, and no one has control over how long it lasts. Reasoning with a person (or oneself) about how much time has passed or how to look at the situation rationally doesn't quicken the process.

Hospice continued to call me every month and send new booklets along with letters that described what Earl and I might be going though, and this continued to be very reassuring. The Bereavement Coordinator continued to coach me that it *really was okay* if Earl didn't finish seventh grade Algebra by June. Whatever grieving could be done while the feelings were front and center was way more important than stuffing them away and trying to get back to "business as usual." Even if Earl didn't appear to "be productive" there was a lot going on deep inside. He found some value in talking with his counselor. Whenever he felt like talking, I took time to listen, but I didn't expect him to verbalize what he was going through. Much of the processing was non-verbal. He found it was hard to talk with friends about the death; if a person hadn't been through this, they didn't know what to say, were uncomfortable talking about it, or would change the subject. Some walks and talks with his sisters helped. Rhia could certainly relate. Now and then the two of them would go off on walks together. (She moved back to the area and got a job at a small animal clinic while contemplating graduate school.) It warmed my heart to know that they had each other to grieve with and to remember their dad. Ella could also relate; her beloved mentor, Moe, died at the end of the April.

Earl found chiropractic and cranial-sacral adjustments helped him feel more balanced and calm. It's fortunate that his summer vacation was just around the bend.

I found that Reiki and acupuncture help remind my body how to relax, to not be hypervigilant all the time. We were lucky to live in a place with many professional healers, and I was fortunate to have friends who offered me various kinds of body work. Talking with friends who shared the same spiritual practice also helped. I also found stability in going back to my seasonal cleaning work and working on this book whenever I could; I wanted so much to see it and hold it in my hands that I had to keep on creating it!

Every time Earl came into my room there would be drawings, paintings, and photos all over the place. At first I was worried that all those images would trigger him into sadness or depression, but in fact they were useful as conversation starters. We talked about his dad almost every day. It was a relief to be free to share our memories openly, and we also shared a lot of laughs—even about things I thought he would be offended by, such as my critique of the way his dad used to dress and how lenient he was as a parent. The return of Earl's laughter and his wry sense of humor was another sign of healing.

He enjoyed getting some consolation prizes. Two friends gave him beautiful stones. One of his "fairy Godmothers" sent him a fifty dollar bill with a note: "Time to do something fun! This is *not* for your college fund!"

"Mom, I know this might not sound like a fun thing to you, but can I buy a suit jacket to wear to my cousin's graduation? I've always wanted one like Dad's."

Steve—not a dad substitute, but an ally—explained about the difference between a suit jacket and a blazer, and helped him find the best fit. On sale it cost exactly fifty dollars.

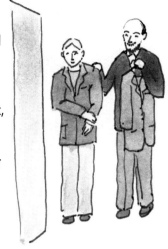

I was trying to figure out a respectful way to tell Earl that I hoped he wouldn't ever wear a hooded sweatshirt under it, but he beat me to the punch. "Don't worry, I won't wear a hooded sweatshirt under it like Dad used to!" We remembered Aubrey's unique style with fondness: the sweatshirt, the suit jacket (even on hikes), the scarf, and always those shades!

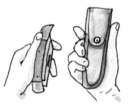

I also gave Earl the money from the sale of the Dad Chair, and told him to spend it in any way he wished.

"Can I get a new carving knife?" he asked.
"Sure, that can be a memento of this time."
"As in: sorry your life sucks, here's a knife?"
"Umm, yeah, I guess."

He went on to joke about the fact that here he was, a teen-aged boy, spending lots of time alone, feeling dejected, and here I was offering to let him buy *a knife*? Was that such a good idea? The fact that we were joking about it and that he valued carving and being creative made it fine. We volleyed a lot of dark humor around. It felt great to laugh. It was important for us to recognize humor, happiness, and pleasure when they naturally arose. We learned it was normal and okay if all these feelings were mixed in together. Just because we were grieving didn't mean we couldn't have fun, and just because we had fun didn't mean we were done with grieving.

Gone but Not Forgotten

On Aubrey's birthday, June 9th, we were going to join Rhia, Anu, and others in the family to spread his ashes, but it was too rainy and windy. Instead we took a walk and had a lovely dinner at Anu's house. She served the famous Dad Salad (on the flowered platter) and broiled salmon with minced garlic, as he used to make it. That intimate candle-lit gathering felt just right.

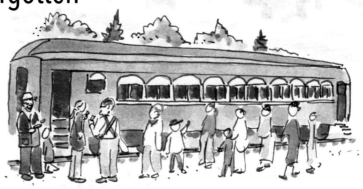

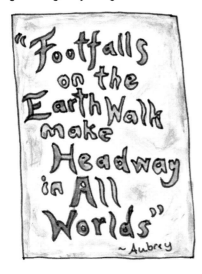

The next day Grand Pops took Earl on a train ride. It ran along a restored section of track that Earl used to walk on with his dad.

In July I hosted a casual gathering at my house. Thinking back to memorial events in which Aubrey and I had participated, I tried to make it something he would have liked to attend: a "celebration of life" but without any formal ceremony. In the corner of the living room near the bookshelf, where all the condolence cards were displayed, I hung some photos of him and a big sheet of plain paper. On a table nearby there were sticky notes and markers so people could write memories and tell us how they knew him. Some guests knew each other and Aubrey better than they knew Earl and me. It was interesting to learn more about him and to read what they wrote on the little notes. Anu brought the quote of his that she had beautifully painted.

Later in the year, Earl and Ella finally had time and interest to see what Mumsie had been working on for months: sorting, labeling, organizing, and archiving old family photographs and old-fashioned clothing. Earl made her day by realizing the connection between the baby in the photograph (who was wearing a long white christening gown), the actual gown, and himself.

"Hey! That baby was really a *real person*! She grew up and had children, and one child was you, and you had my mom, and now *I'm* here - all because that person from long ago *really lived*!"

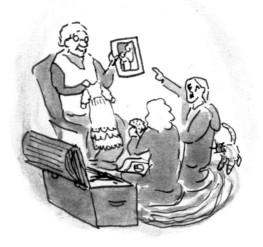

Camp Without Aubrey

Summer was when Earl spent the most time with his dad. I would drop him off at the hiking camp in the morning to take the bus with the campers and go on a hike with his dad. Often he'd stay for the Tuesday and Thursday picnic dinners and go swimming and canoeing at the lake. Over the years I joined them for some picnics, so I knew a few of the campers. A new group came every week throughout the summer, so it was hard for me to keep track of all their names. Aubrey, however, knew everyone. They were like an "extended family" to him. Some had known him for almost thirty years; he'd watched their children grow up and bring their own families to camp. And they, likewise, had watched his children grow up.

One day Earl and I got a call inviting us to come to that evening's picnic. There would also be a casual memorial circle. We knew it would bring up a lot of feelings, but we marshaled our courage and accepted the invitation. Coming around the bend in the driveway where the school bus was parked, we couldn't help but scan its front window for Aubrey.

The picnic and memorial were wonderful. People were so loving, welcoming, and comforting. From the stories they shared we could hear what a huge part of their camp experience Aubrey's presence had been. He'd taken time to listen to their thoughts and have deep conversations. He had often casually hiked alongside the crew members, and helped them carry the lemonade on the all-day hike. That week, one of the new crew members had gone off on the wrong path, and hadn't met the campers at the top of the mountain for lunch. When a safety review meeting was conducted back at camp headquarters, the formal reason written on the report of the incident was, "Aubrey wasn't there to help." Many people still felt his presence amidst the mountains, cabins, and pines. We did too.

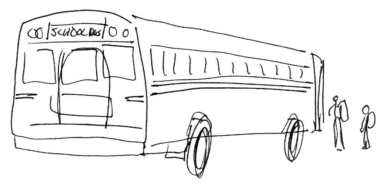

205

Final Reflections

Aubrey's niece mailed us a package of real treasures: baby pictures and photos from his childhood. As with his own photo albums, there are images of people, places, and eras of his life about which I know nothing. Even a whole book about a person only scratches the surface of who they really are. Each of us is a mystery, made up of so many details. There are moments when we become aware of this mystery: meeting a newborn baby, falling in love, reflecting on someone after they have gone. Even after a person dies we may learn new things about them and expand our perception of who they were.

~

In Aubrey's plain leather wallet there were $6.00, a photo of his daughter, a credit card, a debit card, a national park pass, and four library cards.

~

Aubrey willed his car to his mechanic as an "organ donor." When the guy came to tow the car, he told me Aubrey had always paid him, eventually. "Never had anyone try so hard to do things right," he said.

~

The dramas Aubrey and I went through were never the point of our relationship. If he'd always made it easy for me to love him, I'd only have learned to practice conditional love; "I love you because you deserve it." But, no matter what we went through, love would transcend the problems; I would feel my heart opening again, regardless of the circumstances. He, more than anyone, helped me learn about and experience the reality of unconditional love.

~

This fall my first ex-husband, The Gardener, wins the prize for generosity above and beyond the call of duty. Seeing Earl moping about, and Ella on leave from college, sad and upset about putting her life on hold, he offered them the gift of travel. The three of them went on a two week camping trip to the Grand Canyon and other monumental landscapes of the Southwest. Earl came home uplifted, more confident, with refreshed enthusiasm for life.

While they were away I focused on writing this last chapter. I also stayed home to take care of Tucker, who turned a corner into declining health. Seven months (to the day) after Aubrey died, Tucker crossed over as well. We all miss him dearly; he was a sweet, joyful, and loving pup throughout his life.

~

Now that it's November, trees are nearly bare. This was the season, a year ago, that the Dad Walks turned into Study Hall. As snow begins to fall, memories of the past winter are coming back into view. We'll have to get used to Aubrey's absence through a whole new batch of seasonal associations. Family holidays are some of the hardest times for those who have recently lost a loved one. What will it be like to watch *The Polar Express* without Dad, Earl wonders? I told him I can still make cocoa with marshmallows. Thanksgiving dinner will be at our house this year, with Mumsie and Gandpops, Ella and her dad, Steve, Earl, and me around the dining room table. A festive celebration will do this house some good!

~

This final story is shared for fun–but with apologies to one of Aubrey's hiking camp friends–I hope you will laugh with us!

Aubrey used to comment on my handwriting: How could someone who tried to be as in-control as I did have such messy handwriting? Earl wondered the same thing, and was often critical of the notes I'd jot on his schoolwork. How bad was it? Well: when I mailed the obituary to each person who'd sent a check by mail, I included a little card in each envelope thanking them for the amount of their donation. One person wrote back a thank you for that thank you, and said that she would cherish the note, "scribbled by Aubrey in his dying hand." So now we know, for a fact: my handwriting is as bad as that of a dying man. Earl and I laughed so hard about this that tears streamed down our faces and we got stitches in our bellies–but in a good way. ✍

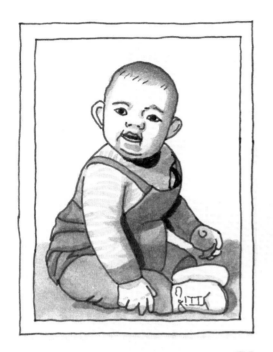
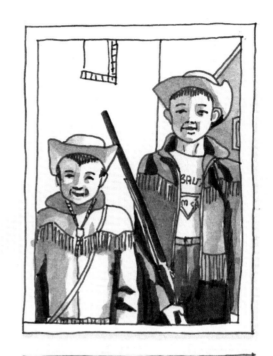
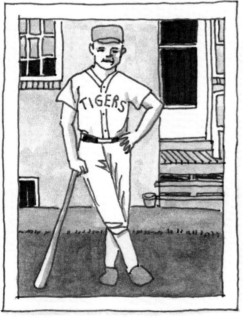
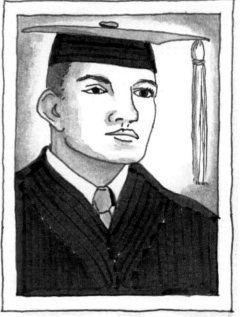

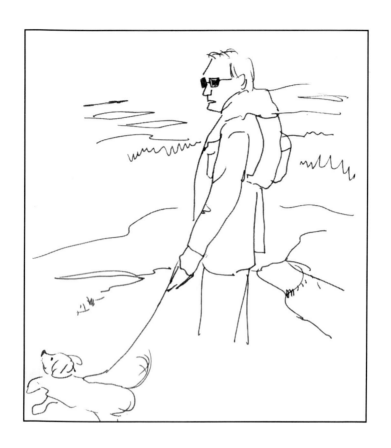

Aubrey Jameson Bart

June 9, 1949 - April 16, 2017

Tucker Shiloh

February 14, 2004 - November 16, 2017

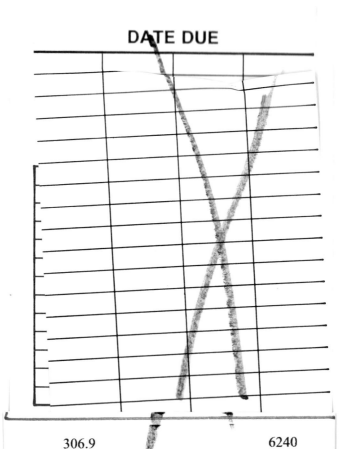